HEALTHY THERMO COOKING
for Busy Families

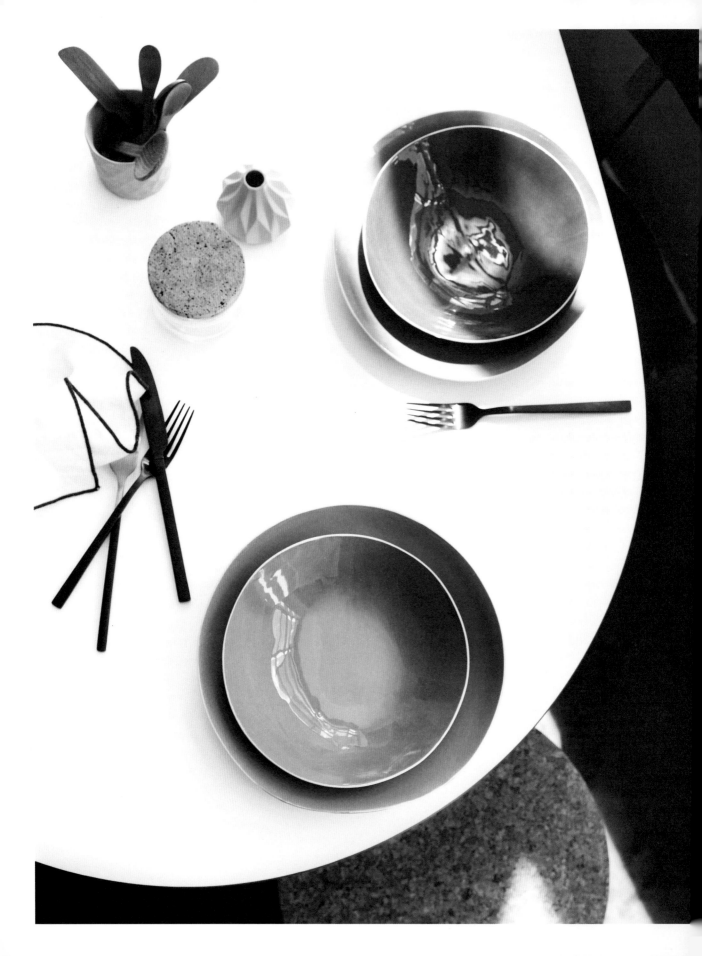

HEALTHY THERMO COOKING
for Busy Families

OLIVIA ANDREWS

MURDOCH BOOKS
SYDNEY · LONDON

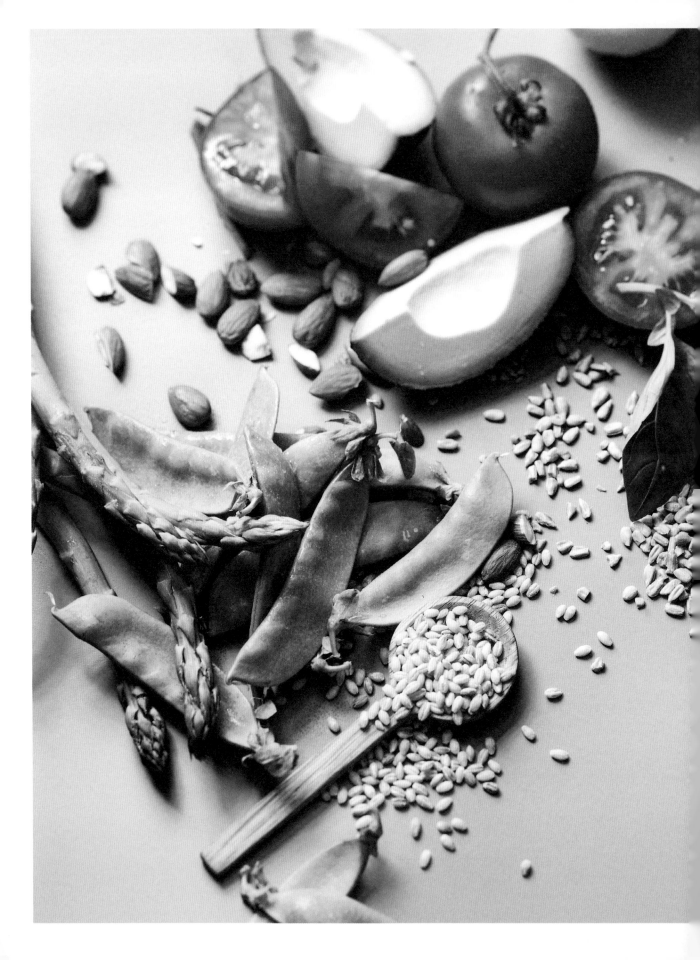

CONTENTS

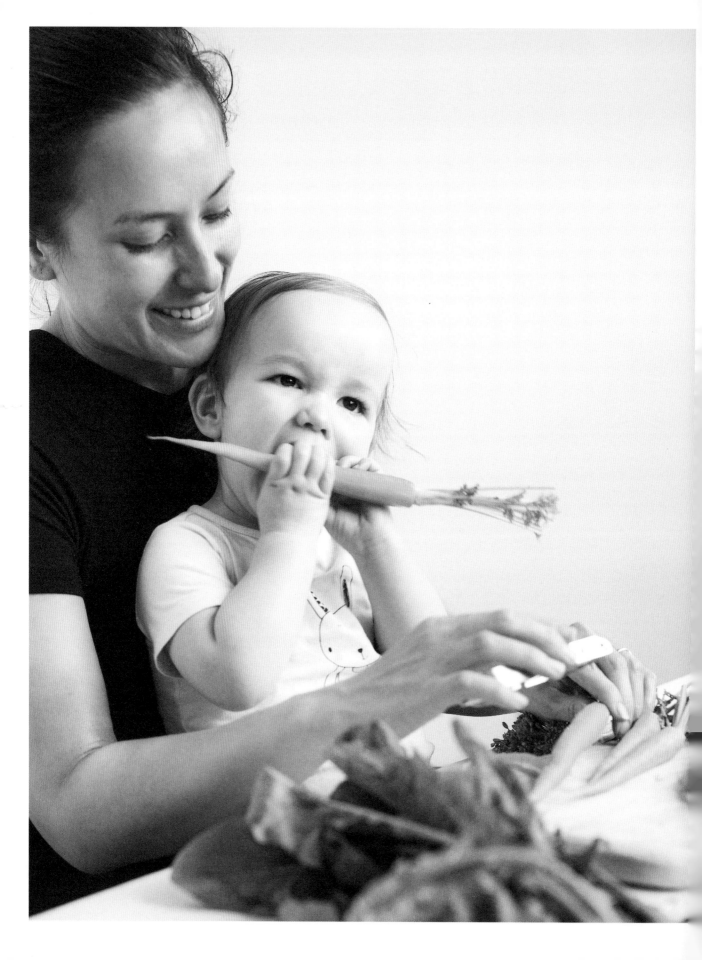

INTRODUCTION

Day-to-day life is hectic, and just when you think things can't possibly get busier, they do. Like most parents, I want my family to eat well and feel good, and making sure we all get the best possible nutrition plays on my mind. But the daily juggle can make chasing a perfectly 'healthy' diet tricky – it often feels unachievable or more inaccessible than it should, be it due to cost of ingredients, lack of time or because you're navigating the ever-changing preferences of fussy eaters. Cooking smarter and faster is the only way I am able to strike some sort of balance between time pressures and health. When I finally came around to the idea of buying a thermo device, I fell hard. These all-in-one appliances can be a gift in the kitchen and a valuable tool for a busy family. The extent to which a thermo device can become a part of everyday family life is quite extraordinary – the magnitude of what you can achieve with this compact piece of equipment is nothing short of genius.

I cook for a living, but even so I often find myself wondering how I managed before I owned a thermo. This may sound a little over-the-top but my thermo device really has changed the way mealtimes operate in my household. It alleviates so much of the workload of cooking a meal; it weighs ingredients, chops, grates and blends them, then cooks and steams them to perfection. But, for me, the real freedom comes from being able to leave it to get on with stirring and cooking while I do other things. And at the end of the meal, we aren't left with a stack of dirty dishes and pans to deal with. No drama! Not only has it changed the way we do things, we also feel much lighter and better on the inside now that there's less frying (oils don't get anywhere near the smoking point they do when frying), and steaming is now the norm.

There's no denying that some brands of thermo devices can be expensive, but I treat mine as an investment in our household. In the long run, our lifestyle, well-being *and* bank balance are better off. I make a heap of pantry staples as I need them, and you might find this is something that works for your family too. Whether that means milling your own flours, making your own milk, bread, butter, spreads or condiments – your thermo can do it all. When I make these simple essentials, not only are they more nutritious than their supermarket equivalents because they're made from whole, fresh ingredients, they also get a far better response from my family. By making these staples in smaller amounts as needed, you'll hopefully find you throw out far less food. Less waste is always a good thing.

As great as all of these benefits are, perhaps the greatest benefit is the way we are able to plan ahead. Batch cooking is where my thermo really comes into its own, whether it be cooking something a day ahead or 3 months in advance. Next to a thermo device, I'd say a freezer is one of the greatest allies a busy family can have (OK, and a dishwasher). Let those two things join forces and you'll achieve next-level organisation. I've noted whenever a meal freezes well, which happens to be for the majority of the recipes in the book. One of the best pieces of advice I can give you is that if you can fit a double batch in your device, do it! Driving home on a busy day knowing you have a freezer full of healthy meals that only need reheating feels amazing.

The recipes have been carefully thought out and created for cooks of any level, from beginners to avid thermo users alike. You'll find many classics and family favourites, plenty of traditional kids' recipes (adapted and suitable for big kids too!) and a few exciting new combinations to try – all with a healthy twist. I've snuck in as much goodness and as many vegetables as I possibly can, hopefully in a way that no one feels like they're missing out.

There are simple sauces you'll use again and again, as well as complete meals where the protein element, grains AND veggies are all cooked in the thermo at the same time. This may seem ambitious, but I promise that once you start using your device this way, and cooking all the elements together, it will become a no-brainer.

The Everyday Basics chapter includes some of my favourite go-to ingredients, like a great all-round pasta sauce, homemade butter, yoghurt and labne, and nut butters so delicious they should come with a warning label. You can make the base recipe for many of them, then turn them into other delightful staples to store in the fridge, freezer or cupboard. It's well worth making them up in advance for use later on. I've used most of these basics in recipes throughout the book, but you can swap in store-bought equivalents if you haven't had time to whip them up.

Recipes that are quick, easy, healthy, nutritious, delicious and family-friendly are what we want, so the Super Soups and Weeknight Wonders chapters have been designed to tick every box. Using a thermo device means you'll barely need to lift a finger, except to direct the kids to the table. The majority of the recipes in the Slower Dinners chapter can be made ahead and frozen. These ones are great for weekend cook-ups that include the whole family or for preparing if you've got some really busy weeks coming up.

You might be surprised to discover that your device can also churn out many more desserts beyond ice creams and sorbets. The Sweet Somethings chapter has a good range of yummy desserts, all of which use natural sugars (or offer alternatives) in much lower quantities than traditional recipes might use. There are even a few guilt-free dessert options too.

All in all, different things work for different families. Whatever your situation, I hope you enjoy cooking these recipes for your family. You now have the device, the information and the ability to create an endless amount of one-bowl wonders.

Here's to happy and healthy thermo cooking, everyone!

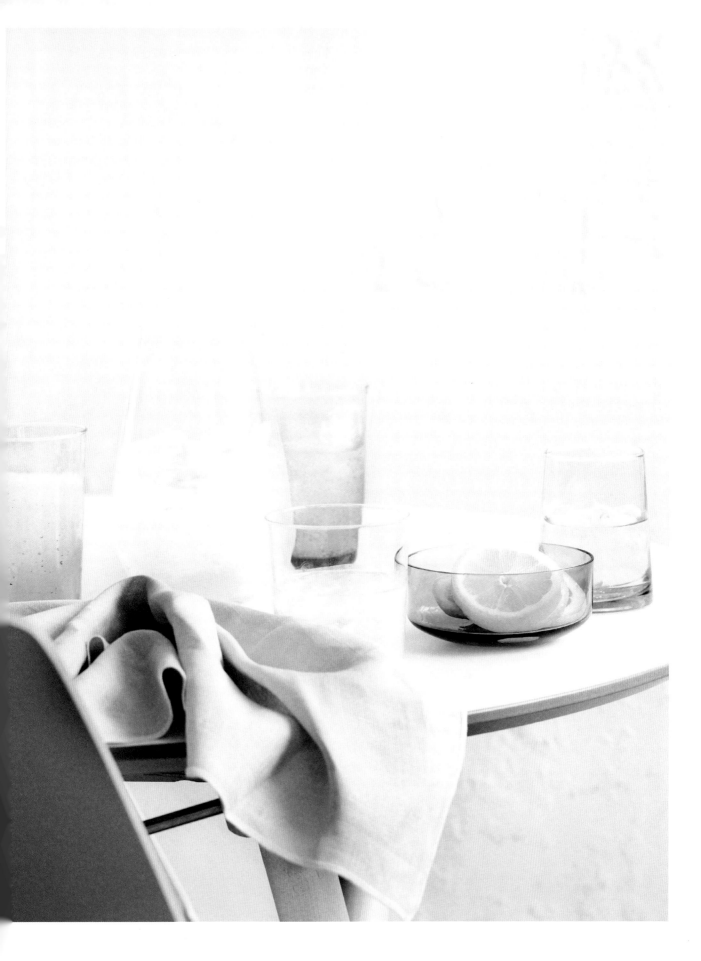

INGREDIENTS

▶ **Flours and nutmeals**

Because I suffer from eczema and have a moderate sensitivity to gluten, I've had to rethink how I approach recipes, and how I cook in general. Since gluten sensitivity is an issue for many, you'll find that about 75% of the recipes in this book are gluten-free, and that I also offer alternatives and suggestions for making things gluten-free wherever possible. My gut thanks me for using wholewheat organic flour, and I mill my own in the thermo whenever I need it. It's honestly so quick and easy to make your own nutmeals and flours, you won't look back.

▶ **Meat**

If meat plays a major role in your meals, you might notice that these recipes call for less meat than you're used to using. As a society, we eat far more meat or animal fats than we ever used to – we certainly don't need to eat meat every day to maintain a healthy diet. And while we often hear we should consume certain foods and drinks in moderation, this message is not as clear when it comes to meat. I prefer to use smaller quantities of meat, and bulk up dishes with lots of other good stuff, like veggies and wholegrains. That way, I still get the flavour and texture, but with the added bonus of it being more cost-effective and nutritious.

Cooking less meat also means that you don't have to skimp on quality. I buy good-quality meat, be it free-range, organic or grass-fed. I find this to be the best solution for my family, but everybody is different. If you prefer to include more meat in your family meals, simply bump up the amount called for in a recipe by 100 g (3½ oz).

▶ **Dairy**

My family responds well to yoghurt and white cheeses, which is great because yoghurt can be used in place of many dairy products that are high in saturated fats, like sour cream and cream cheese. Just making that simple swap is much better for you. If your family is anything like mine, they probably go through a pretty shocking amount of yoghurt over the course of a week. Making your own dairy products is so easy, very satisfying and can also be cost-effective over the long term.

▶ **Sugar**

Let's not forget our old 'friend' sugar. Sure, you'll find the odd teaspoon of sugar (in its various forms) in recipes throughout the book. I feel it's important to balance flavours within a dish, but its use is never too excessive and you know exactly how much you're putting in. I've also offered alternatives to processed sugar where possible and you'll likely find the sweetness in the recipes is noticeably lower than what you may be used to.

▶ **Fresh herbs**

Fresh herbs are a must have in my kitchen. Not only are they fantastic flavour additions, but they are really nutritious too. When I include coriander (cilantro), parsley or dill in a recipe, you'll notice that I often include the stems. I usually chop the stems of these herbs with the other ingredients, as they're perfectly good to use, plus there's less waste (and the hassle of picking them is bypassed). Stems have more flavour than the leaves and add texture too.

▶ **Fruit and veggies**

In a perfect world, I'd buy organic everything if I could, but most of the time, it's just not feasible or affordable. The good news is that you can get away with buying non-organic fruits and vegetables, like oranges or pumpkin (winter squash), if you plan on peeling their skins anyway. But for ingredients that you plan on eating in their entirety, like blueberries, leafy greens, herbs or broccoli, it's great to buy organic, if you can. Either way, always give your fruit and vegetables a good wash before you prepare them.

Salt

I believe that seasoning your food throughout the cooking process is imperative. I'm not talking about using bucket loads, or any old table salt. For me, it has to be natural sea salt. Of course when we're cooking for kids we need to be careful about how much we add because their little kidneys can't process salt like ours can. But that's one of the best things about cooking for your family – you have full control over how much salt is added to your food. Seasoning with a pinch here and there from the beginning of the cooking process helps to unlock the flavours of your ingredients, and it's a drop in the ocean compared to the high levels of (bad) sodium found in processed foods, especially in lots of kids' foods on supermarket shelves.

USING YOUR THERMO DEVICE

These are a few pointers you may find useful when cooking your way through this book:

Timings vary from device to device

It's good to remember that there are slight variations in the cooking results between the various thermo devices on the market. Wherever relevant and possible, I have included a cooking time as well as the result to look out for to help account for the differences in thermo devices. For example, if vegetables aren't tender in the cooking time I've suggested, continue to cook them until they are tender and you achieve the desired result. The same applies if something is done to your liking – there's no need to continue cooking. Feel free to make recipes work for you, and tweak the timings according to how your device deals with them.

Rinsing between steps

Don't worry about washing out your jug in between steps unless absolutely necessary.

I've generally ordered the method to allow for this, leaving some flavours in the jug will only add flavour to the final product. That's no bad thing!

Chopping vegetables

When roughly chopping vegetables, don't worry too much about size. Just don't chop the veggies too small. The blades in your mixer bowl will pulverise the ingredients in no time, so you are only cutting them in order to fit them into the bowl. A good guide is an average carrot – I would chunk it into thirds or quarters before adding it to my device.

Sterilising jars

Particularly in the basics section, I suggest using sterilised jars, which is yet another thing you can use your brilliant device for. Just add 500 g (1 lb 2 oz) of water to the mixer bowl then place the clean jars and their lids upside down on your steaming tray. Sterilise them for **20 min/120°C/speed 1**, then move the tray to the counter and fill with the ingredient you are storing.

Heat-processing (AKA 'bottling')

If you want to store the sauces and condiments longer than the 3 months I've suggested in the recipes, you can make them even more stable with 'heat-processing'. This works well for pasta sauces, relishes, jams and chutneys. (There are lots of how-to guides online if you want a detailed walk through the process.) Place a rack or tea towel on the bottom of large saucepan or stock pot then stand the filled and sterilised glass jars upright on top, so they aren't touching the bottom of the pan. Pour in enough hot water to cover the jars by 2.5 cm (1 in). Place over a low–medium heat and bring to a gentle simmer (don't let it boil) for 30 minutes. Top up with more hot water, if needed. Use tongs to remove the jars to a heatproof surface, cool completely then label and store in a cool, dark cupboard for up to one year, unopened.

EVERYDAY BASICS

NAKED PASTA SAUCE

Making your own tomato sauce is a great way of putting an abundance of tomatoes to good use at the height of the season, when they're especially ripe and sweet. This sauce is the most used recipe in the book, so keeping it 'naked' and pure allows you to use it in a whole variety of dishes and cuisines.

MAKES APPROXIMATELY 1.25 LITRES (44 FL OZ/5 CUPS)
Preparation time 10 minutes
Cooking time 30 minutes

1.5 kg (3 lb 5 oz) very ripe roma (plum) tomatoes
2 garlic cloves
4 tablespoons extra virgin olive oil
2 teaspoons fine sea salt
raw, white or caster (superfine) sugar, to taste

Add the maximum amount of water that can be boiled in the mixer bowl and bring to the boil for **5 min/100°C/speed 2,** or until the water boils. Meanwhile, using a small sharp knife, score a cross at the top and bottom of each tomato and place them into a large heatproof bowl.

Pour the boiling water over the tomatoes so they are completely submerged then set aside for 30 seconds, or until their skins start to split. Drain and rinse under cold running water to cool then remove and discard the skins. If not all of the skins come off, just leave them on.

Blend the peeled tomatoes and garlic for **10 sec/speed 5**. Scrape down the side of the bowl. Add the oil and salt. Cook for **25 min/100°C/speed 1**. If necessary, add sugar to taste.

Pour the hot sauce into warm sterilised jars (see page 11) with airtight lids and seal. Turn the jars upside down on a heatproof surface and leave to cool. Store the sauce in a cool, dark place for up to 3 months. Once opened, keep refrigerated for up to 1 week or freeze for up to 6 months.

See photograph on page 16.

MAKE AHEAD: PANTRY | FRIDGE | FREEZER
GLUTEN-FREE | NUT-FREE | PALEO | VEGAN

TIP
I use roma tomatoes as they are meatier and have fewer seeds, but feel free to use vine-ripened if you prefer. The sweetness of the tomatoes, depends on their ripeness, so you can add sugar to taste, starting with half a teaspoon at a time.

PIZZA SAUCE

I've struggled to find a pizza sauce recipe that I really love, until now. This is the perfect balance between fresh and rich, and it's a good one to have on hand in your pantry, fridge or freezer. Your mixer can easily handle a quadruple batch, and that is well worth doing. Once made, you can use this on the Cauliflower pizzas (page 123), or as the sauce for a traditional pizza using the dough recipe on page 138.

MAKES APPROXIMATELY 185 ML (6 FL OZ/¾ CUP)

Preparation time 5 minutes
Cooking time 10 minutes

400 g (14 oz) Naked pasta sauce (opposite page)
  or tinned chopped tomatoes
2 tablespoons tomato paste (concentrated purée)
1 teaspoon dried oregano
1 handful basil leaves (optional)

Add all of the ingredients to the mixer bowl and cook for **10 min/120°C/ speed 1**.

Spoon the hot sauce into a warm sterilised jar (see page 11) with an airtight lid and seal. Turn the jar upside down on a heatproof surface and leave to cool.

Store the sauce in a cool, dark place for up to 3 months. Once opened, keep refrigerated for up to 1 week or freeze for up to 6 months.

See photograph on page 17.

MAKE AHEAD: PANTRY | FRIDGE | FREEZER
GLUTEN-FREE | NUT-FREE | PALEO | VEGAN

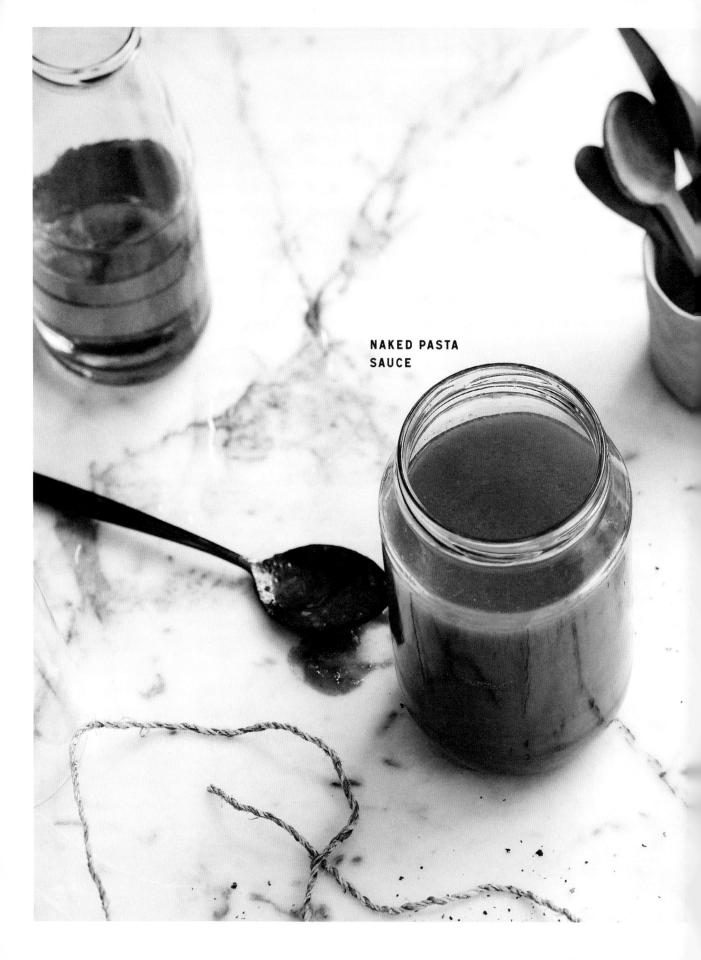

NAKED PASTA
SAUCE

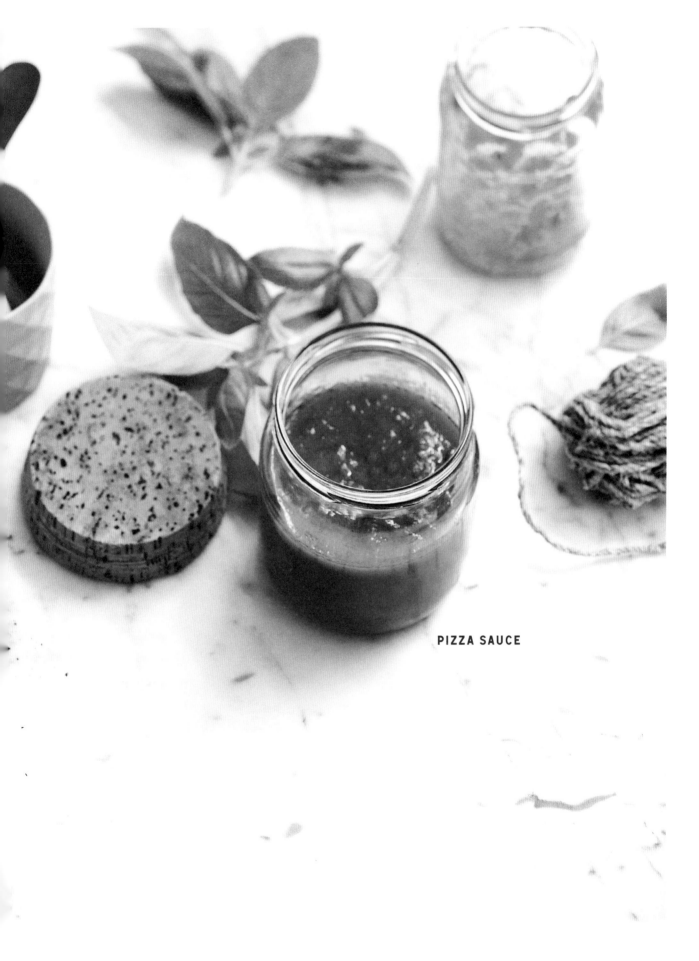

PIZZA SAUCE

TOMATO AND CAPSICUM RELISH

The amount of sugar in a typical store-bought relish can be off the charts. In this relish, natural sweetness (as well as goodness) comes from the capsicum, apple and the red onion. This can be enjoyed hot or cold, and served with many different dishes as a substitute for tomato sauce.

MAKES APPROXIMATELY 500 G (1 LB 2 OZ)

Preparation time 5 minutes
Cooking time 25 minutes

1 red capsicum (pepper), stem and seeds removed, roughly chopped
1 apple, peeled, cored and quartered
1 red onion, peeled and quartered
250 ml (9 fl oz/1 cup) Naked pasta sauce (page 14) or tinned chopped tomatoes
125 ml (4 fl oz/½ cup) maple syrup or 4 tablespoons raw, white or caster (superfine) sugar
185 ml (6 fl oz/¾ cup) red wine vinegar
1½ teaspoons fine sea salt

Blend the capsicum, apple and onion for **6 sec/speed 5**. Scrape down the side of the bowl.

Add all of the remaining ingredients. Cook for **25 min/120°C/speed 2**.

Pour the hot mixture into a warm sterilised jar (see page 11) with an airtight lid and seal. Turn the jar upside down on a heatproof surface and leave to cool.

Store the relish in a cool, dark place for up to 6 months. Once opened, keep refrigerated for up to 1 month.

MAKE AHEAD: PANTRY | FRIDGE
DAIRY-FREE | GLUTEN-FREE | NUT-FREE | PALEO | VEGAN

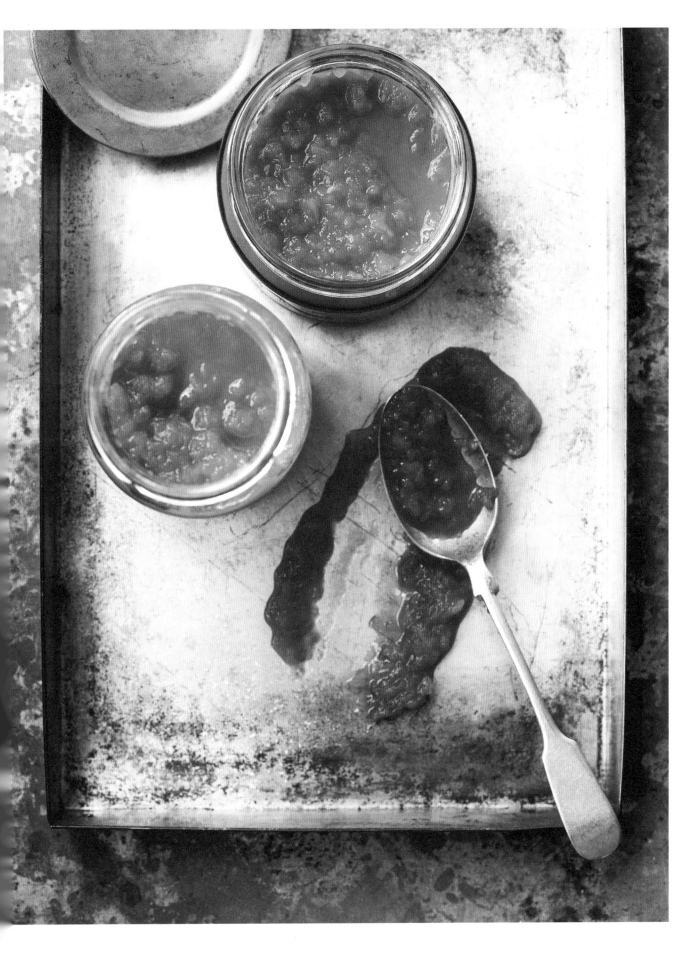

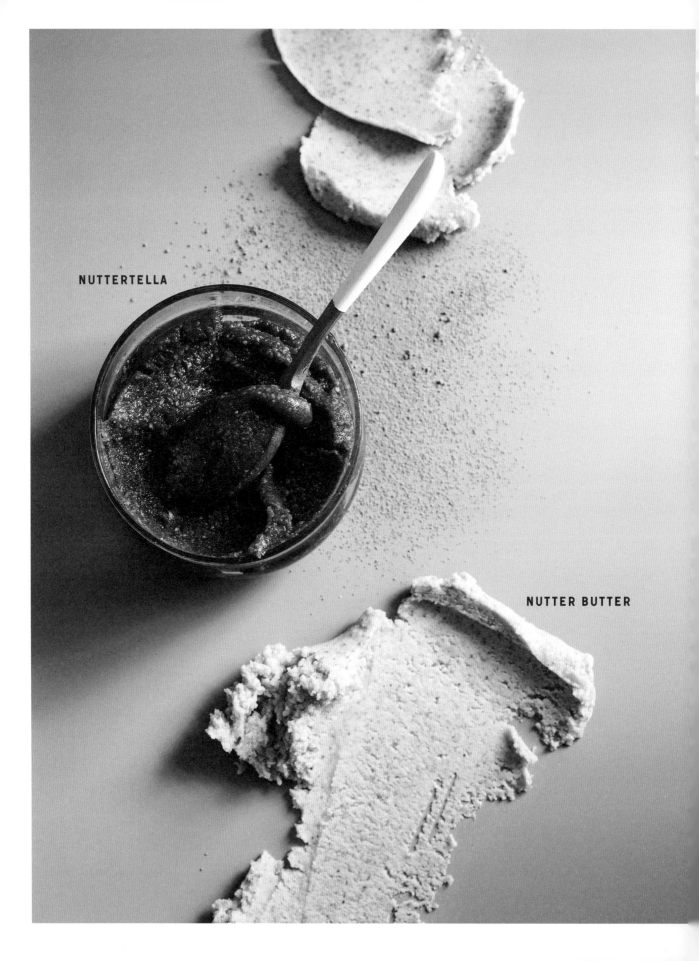

NUTTERTELLA

NUTTER BUTTER

NUTTER BUTTER

Homemade nut butters are crazy good! I like to make mine with a blend of macadamia and cashews, but you can use your favourite variety or a blend, and vary the proportions here. The higher the fat content of the nuts, the creamier the result. If I'm planning to use half of the batch for the Nuttertella (see right), I use cashews, macadamias and hazelnuts in a 1:1:3 ratio.

MAKES 500 G (1 LB 2 OZ)
Preparation time 5 minutes

100 g (3½ oz) cashews
100 g (3½ oz) macadamias
300 g (10½ oz) almonds (or skinless hazelnuts, if using to make Nuttertella)
¼ teaspoon fine sea salt
1 tablespoon olive oil or grapeseed oil (optional)

Blend the nuts and salt for **1 min/speed 9**. Scrape down the side of the bowl. Blend for **1 min/speed 7**, slowly adding the oil if the mixture is too thick.

Store in an airtight container in the fridge for up to 2 weeks.

MAKE AHEAD: FRIDGE
DAIRY-FREE | GLUTEN-FREE | PALEO | VEGAN | VEGETARIAN

NUTTERTELLA

I feel much more comfortable giving my family this spread as a substitute for the highly processed alternatives out there – it contains more nutritious nuts than refined sugar *and* there are no hidden nasties. Double the recipe if you would like to have more in the fridge, or if you want to make the mousse or the truffles on page 182.

MAKES 700 G (1 LB 9 OZ)
Preparation time 5 minutes

50 g (1¾ oz) cashews
50 g (1¾ oz) macadamias
150 g (5½ oz) skinless hazelnuts
fine sea salt
2 tablespoons raw cacao powder
4 tablespoons maple syrup

Blend the nuts and a large pinch of sea salt for **1 min/speed 9** until just combined. Scrape down the side of the bowl.

Add the cacao powder and maple syrup and blend for **1 min/speed 7**, or until you have a soft paste. Take care not to overmix and split this – you want a soft homogeneous mixture.

Store in an airtight container in the fridge for up to 2 weeks.

MAKE AHEAD: FRIDGE
DAIRY-FREE | GLUTEN-FREE | PALEO | VEGAN | VEGETARIAN

CULTURED BUTTER AND REAL BUTTERMILK

For me, a generic store-bought block of butter cannot compete with the flavour of this homemade one. Adding a culture to the cream in the form of yoghurt not only improves the flavour, but also makes it easier for your gut to digest.

MAKES APPROXIMATELY 250 G (9 OZ) BUTTER AND 250 ML (9 FL OZ/1 CUP) BUTTERMILK

Preparation time 10 minutes + standing time
Cooking time 2 minutes

600 ml (21 fl oz) thin (pouring/whipping) cream
70 g (2½ oz/3 tablespoons) yoghurt (page 26), pot-set natural
   or Greek-style yoghurt
3 tablespoons fine sea salt

Add the cream and yoghurt to the bowl and cook for **2 min/37°C/ speed 2**, or until the mixture reaches 37°C (99°F). Cover and leave at room temperature for 6 hours, or preferably overnight. Place in the fridge until cold.

Meanwhile, combine the salt with 500 ml (17 fl oz/2 cups) of cold water in a jug and store in the fridge or freezer until very cold.

Insert the whisk attachment. Whisk the mixture for **2–3 min/speed 4** until the butter solids separate from the buttermilk. Pour the milk through a sieve into a jug. Store the milk in an airtight container in the fridge for up to 1 week.

Pour the chilled saltwater solution into the mixer bowl. Whisk for **5 sec/ speed 4**. Pour the water through a sieve and discard. Using very cold hands, gently squeeze out as much excess liquid as possible.

Shape the butter into a log or wheel, wrap up in baking paper and store in the fridge. Best used within 2 weeks.

See photograph on page 24.

MAKE AHEAD: FRIDGE
GLUTEN-FREE | NUT-FREE | VEGETARIAN

TIP
When squeezing out the buttermilk from the butter, run your hands under cold water or rub with ice cubes to ensure they are nice and cold. The more buttermilk you can squeeze out of the butter, the longer the butter will last.

NO-WORK 'SOURDOUGH'

I've tried many different forms of this recipe over the years, and it really doesn't get any easier than making it with my thermo device. It requires next to no work, hence the name!

If using wholewheat grains, mill them for 1 min/speed 10 until ground. You'll get a much denser bread but you'll be retaining a lot of the goodness that gets lost in commercial flour-making. The dough will be very sticky and a bit thicker than a pancake when transferring to the tray, but have faith! It will rise into a beautiful loaf of bread.

MAKES 1 LOAF

Preparation time 5 minutes + standing time
Cooking time 40 minutes

500 g (1 lb 2 oz) wholewheat or plain (all-purpose) flour
2 teaspoons fine sea salt
½ teaspoon raw, white or caster (superfine) sugar
2 teaspoons dried active yeast

Add all of the ingredients to the bowl and pour in 425 g (15 oz) of water. Blend for **1 min/37°C/speed 2**. Transfer to a large bowl and cover with plastic wrap. Refrigerate for at least 6 hours, or preferably overnight.

Take the bowl of dough out of the fridge and leave at room temperature for 30 minutes before baking.

Meanwhile, preheat the oven to 220°C (425°F). Line a tray with baking paper. Using a spatula, carefully transfer the very sticky dough to the lined tray. Gently shape into a round or loaf, but don't touch it too much. However it lands on the tray will be fine.

Bake for 30–40 minutes until the bread is golden and sounds hollow when tapped on the bottom. Set aside to cool for at least 15 minutes before slicing.

Serve with cultured butter (see opposite page).

See photograph on page 25.

NUT-FREE | VEGETARIAN | VEGAN

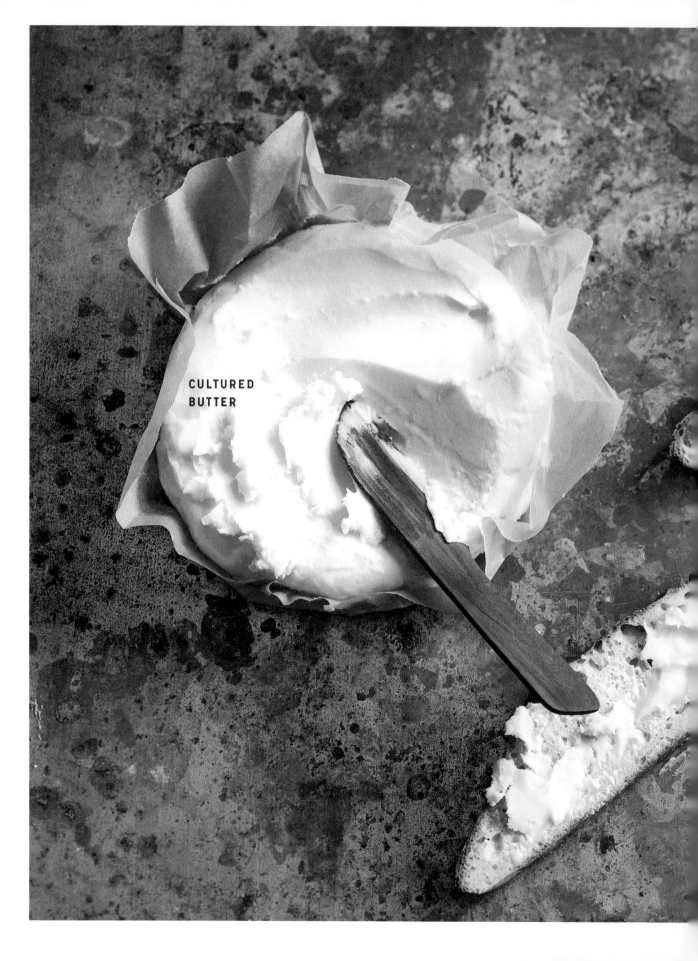

CULTURED
BUTTER

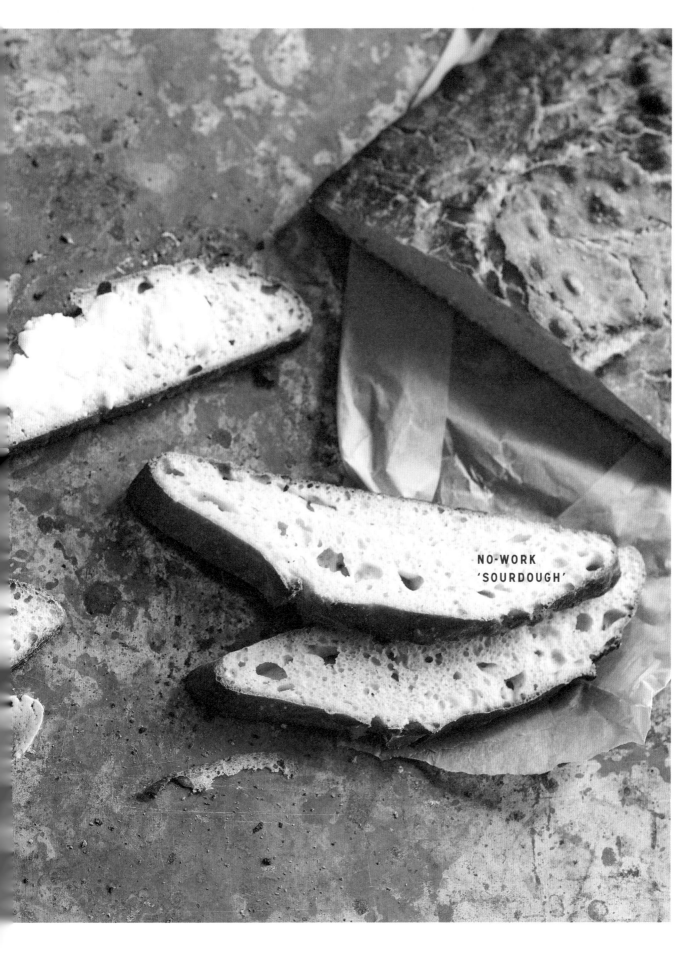

NO-WORK
'SOURDOUGH'

HOMEMADE GOAT'S YOGHURT

When making yoghurt, it's important to heat the milk to just below boiling point (90°C/194°F). This changes the structure of the protein and gives it a better chance of setting. I like using goat's milk for many reasons, but mostly because my family seems to respond better to goat's milk than cow's milk. We also love the taste and the ease of turning that milk into goat's cheese! Goat's milk products are more expensive, but making your own yoghurt can be a great way to save (see Notes).

MAKES 1 KG (2 LB 4 OZ/4 CUPS)
Preparation time 5 minutes + standing time
Cooking time 12 minutes

1 litre (35 fl oz/4 cups) plain goat's milk (see Notes)
3 tablespoons pot-set goat's yoghurt

Add the milk to the bowl and cook for **10 min/90°C/speed 3,** or until the temperature gauge on your device reaches 90°C (194°F). Remove the lid and let the milk to cool to 45°C (113°F). This will take about 40 minutes.

Discard any skin that has formed on the top. Ladle about 250 ml (9 fl oz/1 cup) of the cooled milk into a bowl with the yoghurt and mix well to combine. Add this yoghurt mixture to the mixer bowl and cook for **2 min/speed 2** until the mixture reaches 45°C again.

Meanwhile, warm up one or two hot packs or a hot water bottle. Take out a portable food cooler and two blankets.

Pour the hot mixture into glass sterilised jar(s) (see page 11) with airtight lids, then seal. Sit the jars in the centre of the blankets and place a hot pack or hot water bottle over the top of each lid. Wrap the jars up in the blankets so they are completely covered. Place in the cooler, ensuring the jars are sitting upright. Cover with the lid. Leave for 8–10 hours, or overnight.

Place the jars in the fridge until cold. The yoghurt will keep in the fridge in sealed jars for up to 4 weeks. Once opened, use within 1 week (see Notes).

See photograph on page 28.

MAKE AHEAD: FRIDGE
GLUTEN-FREE | NUT-FREE | VEGETARIAN

NOTES
Once you've made your first batch with store-bought yoghurt, you can reserve 3 tablespoons of your homemade batch to make the next one, and so on.

If you aren't keen on goat's yoghurt, you can just use cow's milk and make cow's yoghurt instead.

LABNE

Out with store-bought processed cream cheese and in with homemade labne! My favourite alternative to cream cheese, this labne tastes so much better and is so much better for you – it has far less sodium and lots more calcium than processed cream cheese.

If you're after a similar flavour profile to cream cheese, cow's yoghurt is the best choice. That said, for the best homemade cheese or curd, goat's labne is incredible. It's such a versatile ingredient and so easy to make. All of the hard work has already been done by your mixer in the yoghurt-making process. This recipe is used as part of other recipes in the book, from sauces to icings, so it's well worth the effort and yet another good trick to have up your sleeve.

MAKES APPROXIMATELY 260 G (9¼ OZ/1 CUP)

Preparation time 5 minutes + standing time

600 g (1 lb 2 oz) Homemade goat's (or cow's) yoghurt (see opposite page)
1 teaspoon fine sea salt

Add the yoghurt and salt to a bowl and mix until well combined. Line a large, fine-mesh sieve with muslin (cheesecloth) or even two layers of paper towel with enough excess overhanging to cover the surface.

Transfer the yoghurt mixture to the cloth and cover the surface. Sit the sieve inside a bowl or jug to collect any liquid. Chill in the fridge for 1–2 days depending on the desired thickness. Discard any liquid.

Store the labne in an airtight container in the fridge for up to 1 week.

See photograph on page 29.

MAKE AHEAD: FRIDGE
GLUTEN-FREE | NUT-FREE | VEGETARIAN

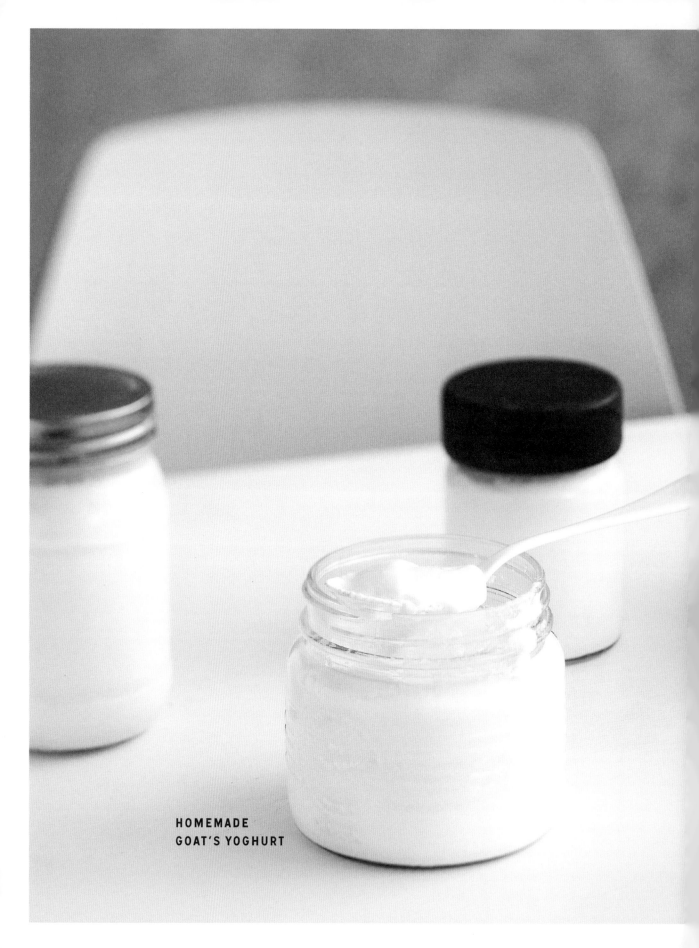

HOMEMADE
GOAT'S YOGHURT

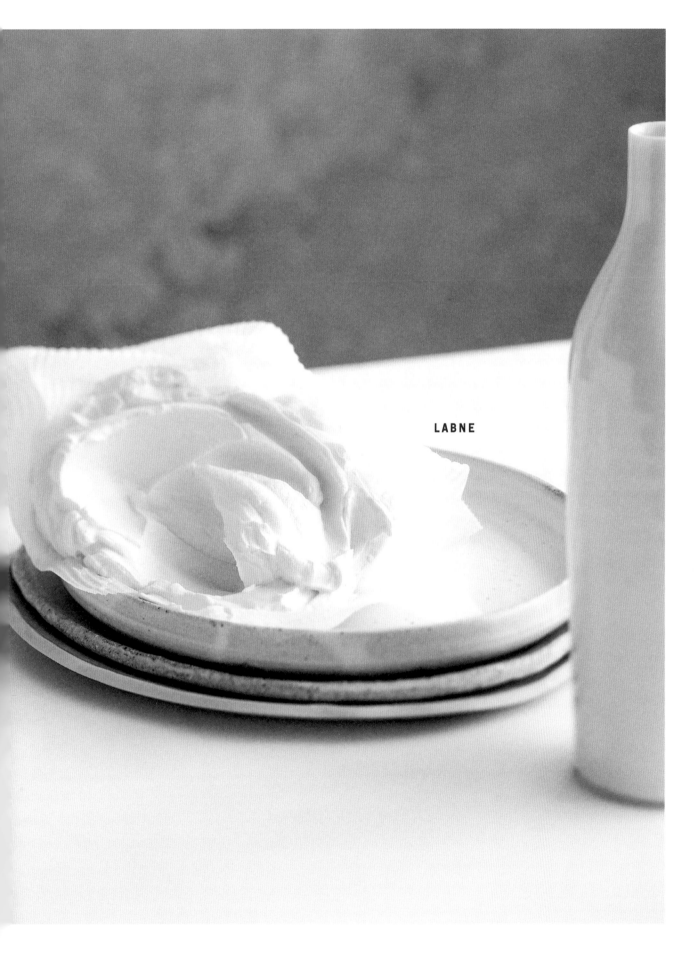

LABNE

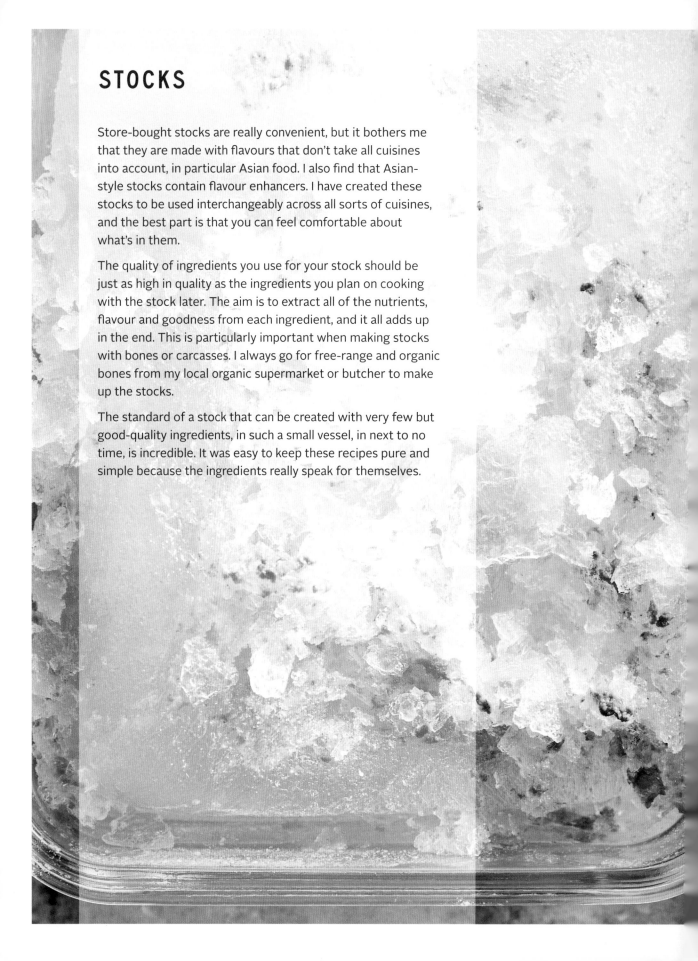

STOCKS

Store-bought stocks are really convenient, but it bothers me that they are made with flavours that don't take all cuisines into account, in particular Asian food. I also find that Asian-style stocks contain flavour enhancers. I have created these stocks to be used interchangeably across all sorts of cuisines, and the best part is that you can feel comfortable about what's in them.

The quality of ingredients you use for your stock should be just as high in quality as the ingredients you plan on cooking with the stock later. The aim is to extract all of the nutrients, flavour and goodness from each ingredient, and it all adds up in the end. This is particularly important when making stocks with bones or carcasses. I always go for free-range and organic bones from my local organic supermarket or butcher to make up the stocks.

The standard of a stock that can be created with very few but good-quality ingredients, in such a small vessel, in next to no time, is incredible. It was easy to keep these recipes pure and simple because the ingredients really speak for themselves.

CHICKEN STOCK

You can make this stock without onion, if you prefer, or you can use brown onion instead of spring onions. Personally, I love the subtlety, flavour and versatility of spring onions. They are also richer in iron, vitamins A and C, calcium and magnesium than your standard onion. Buying the best-quality meat you can afford is important whenever you consume meat, but even more so when boiling the bones to extract all of their goodness. It makes sense that an animal raised under free-range and organic conditions will provide a better quality of nutrients.

MAKES APPROXIMATELY 2 LITRES (70 FL OZ/8 CUPS)
Preparation time 5 minutes
Cooking time 50 minutes

4 spring onions (scallions), roughly chopped
1 chicken carcass, roughly chopped (preferably free-range and organic)
2 teaspoons sea salt (optional)

Chop the onions for **5 sec/speed 5**. Scrape down the side of the bowl. Add the chicken carcass pieces and cook for **10 min/120°C/speed 1**.

Fill the mixer with enough water to reach the capacity line on the inside of the mixer bowl. Add the salt, if using. Cook for **40 min/95°C/speed 1**.

Line a sieve with muslin (cheesecloth) or paper towel then set it inside a large jug. Pour in the stock in batches, discarding any solids.

Store the stock in an airtight container in the fridge for up to 5 days or freeze for up to 6 months.

See photograph on page 35.

MAKE AHEAD: FRIDGE | FREEZER
DAIRY-FREE | GLUTEN-FREE | NUT-FREE | PALEO

VEGETABLE STOCK

Vegetable stocks often lack the richness and intensity of their meat or seafood equivalents. That's why I love adding dried shiitake mushrooms to mine. Their naturally occurring glutamate and full flavour can lift a vegetable stock to a broth reminiscent of a umami-rich meaty stock. Once made, the stock can be used as a base for soups, stews and all sorts of meals. It can also double up as a lovely cleansing hot broth.

MAKES APPROXIMATELY 2 LITRES (70 FL OZ/8 CUPS)
Preparation time 5 minutes + standing time
Cooking time 30 minutes

4 dried shiitake mushrooms
250 ml (9 fl oz/1 cup) boiling water
1 carrot, washed and roughly chopped
1 celery stalk, roughly chopped
2 garlic cloves
5 spring onions (scallions) or 1 leek, washed and roughly chopped
1 teaspoon sea salt (optional)

Put the mushrooms in a jug and pour in the boiling water so they are completely submerged. Cover the jug with a plate and leave to soak for 15 minutes.

Meanwhile, chop the carrot, celery, garlic and spring onions for **3 sec/speed 5**. Scrape down the side of the bowl.

Add the shiitake mushrooms, their soaking liquid and the salt to the mixer bowl. Pour in enough water to reach the capacity line on the inside of your mixer bowl. Cook for **30 min/90°C/speed 1**.

In batches, strain the stock through a fine-mesh sieve set inside a large jug or bowl, discarding the solids.

Store the stock in an airtight container in the fridge for up to 1 week, or freeze for up to 6 months.

See photograph on page 34.

MAKE AHEAD: FRIDGE | FREEZER
DAIRY-FREE | GLUTEN-FREE | NUT-FREE |
PALEO | VEGAN | VEGETARIAN

TIP
Veggie stocks are a great way to use up any vegetables before they are past their best. Don't feel limited to carrots, celery and onions either; corn cobs with their kernels removed give a lovely natural sweetness, and green beans can add a fresh layer of flavour. The options are endless.

SEAFOOD STOCK

This stock can easily be made without any shellfish if there are allergies to consider. I like to use white onion in this stock as it's milder and imparts a cleaner flavour than brown onion. I also use a neutral-tasting oil to ensure the purest fish and seafood flavours come through.

MAKES APPROXIMATELY 2 LITRES (70 FL OZ/8 CUPS)

Preparation time 5 minutes
Cooking time 30 minutes

1 white or brown onion, peeled and halved
2 garlic cloves
1 tablespoon neutral oil, such as grapeseed or rice bran oil
400 g (14 oz) chopped white fish bones, prawn heads and shells
2 teaspoons sea salt (optional)

Chop the onion and garlic for **5 sec/speed 5**. Scrape down the side of the bowl. Add the remaining ingredients and cook for **8 min/120°C/speed 1**.

Fill the mixer with enough water to reach the capacity line on the inside of your mixer bowl.

Cook for **20 min/95°C/speed 1**.

Line a sieve with muslin (cheesecloth) or paper towel and set inside a large jug. In batches, pour in the stock, discarding any solids.

Store the stock in an airtight container in the fridge for up to 3 days, or freeze for up to 3 months.

See photograph on page 35.

MAKE AHEAD: FRIDGE | FREEZER
DAIRY-FREE | GLUTEN-FREE | NUT-FREE | PALEO

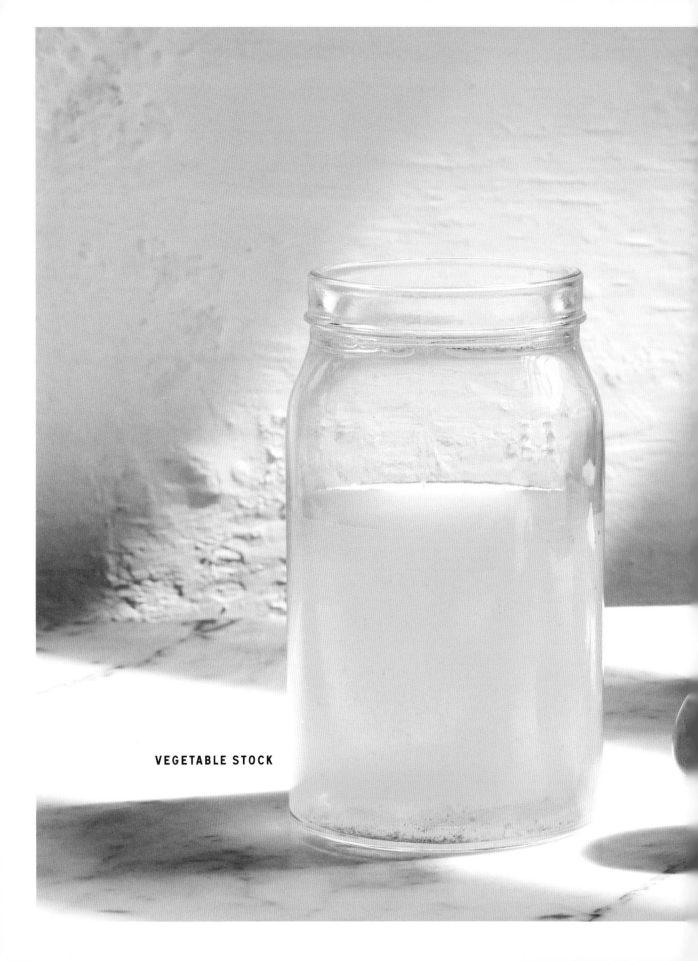

VEGETABLE STOCK

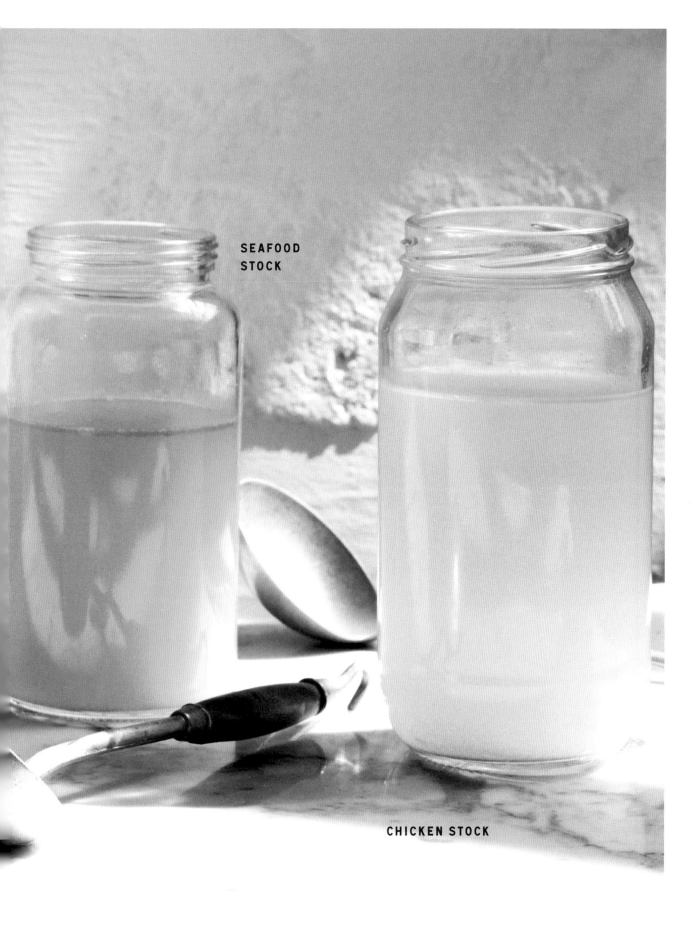

SEAFOOD
STOCK

CHICKEN STOCK

CAULIFLOWER BECHAMEL

I cannot get enough of bechamel. Whatever dish it's in, and whatever the time of day, I just love it. Cauliflower bechamel, however, takes things to a whole new level. The combination of cauliflower and ricotta instead of milk and flour makes this version nearly twice as calcium-rich, astronomically rich in vitamin C *and* a good source of vitamins A and B6. You don't get that from your average bechamel. An added bonus, it's even gluten-free! I top pizzas with it, add it to pasta, put it in moussakas and fish or chicken pie. I even serve it as a simple sauce with meat or fish – it makes everything tastier.

MAKES APPROXIMATELY 600 ML (21 FL OZ)

Preparation time 5 minutes
Cooking time 10 minutes

25 g (1 oz) parmesan cheese (see Note)
75 g (2¾ oz) fontina, provolone or mozzarella cheese
500 g (1 lb 2 oz) cauliflower, roughly chopped
2 garlic cloves
20 g (¾ oz) Butter (page 22) or 1 tablespoon extra virgin olive oil
250 g (9 oz) fresh ricotta cheese

Grate the parmesan for **15 sec/speed 10**. Add the fontina and chop for **8 sec/speed 8**. Transfer to a small bowl.

Chop the cauliflower and garlic for **5 sec/speed 5**. Scrape down the side of the bowl. Add the butter, 250 g (9 oz) of water and season with salt and pepper.

Cook for **8 min/100°C/speed 1**. Blend for **10 sec/speed 8** until smooth. Scrape down the side of the bowl. Next, add the ricotta and the grated cheeses. Cook for **1 min/90°C/speed 3**. Transfer to a bowl, cover and set aside until needed.

Store the bechamel in an airtight container in the fridge and use within 2 days.

MAKE AHEAD: FRIDGE
GLUTEN-FREE | NUT-FREE | VEGETARIAN

NOTE
When cooking for a true vegetarian, keep in mind that some cheeses, including authentic parmesan, are made with calves' rennet. Vegetarian equivalents of these cheeses made with non-animal rennet are widely available in supermarkets and health food stores.

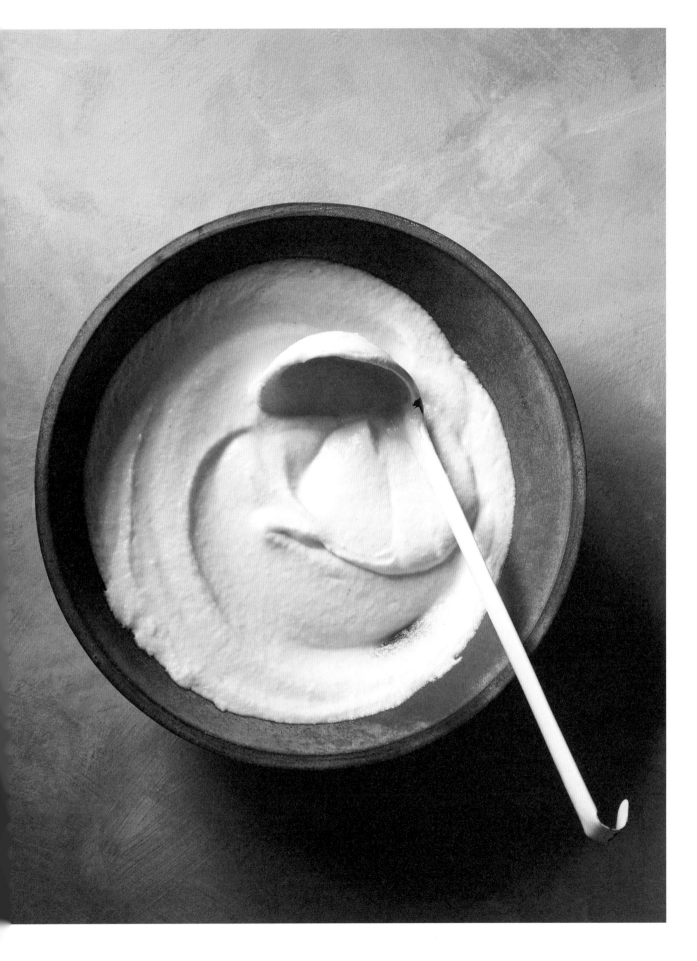

SESAME SEEDS

These tiny seeds are probably up there as one of my all-time favourite ingredients. They may be tiny, but they have enormous benefits, I think they're my ultimate superfood. Sesame seeds are a great source of calcium – there is more calcium in a handful of sesame seeds than in a glass of milk! They are packed with magnesium and iron, and are alkalising too.

When making any of these sesame seed recipes, it's best to start off with raw seeds. Toasted seeds have a shorter shelf life and a very different flavour to freshly toasted seeds. Toast the seeds in a large cold frying pan over medium heat. Stir and shake the pan constantly for 6–8 minutes, until the seeds are evenly golden. Immediately transfer them to the mixer bowl and just omit the first step to warm the seeds.

GOMASIO, THEN TAHINI

Gomasio is a dry Japanese condiment that you can find in Asian supermarkets, but like so many things, it tastes much better when you make your own. I add gomasio to all sorts of dishes, Asian or otherwise. When making gomasio, it's nice if a few whole sesame seeds slip past the blades, so don't worry too much if this happens.

Tahini is a Middle Eastern ingredient best known for being one of the key ingredients in hummus, but it has so many more uses. I often substitute tahini for peanut butter, which makes it a far more versatile ingredient. By adding some oil to the gomasio, you can easily turn it into this fantastically useful ingredient. Because tahini is one of those ingredients that often sits in the fridge for a long time, I prefer making it fresh, and in smaller quantities as and when I need it.

MAKES 125 G (4½ OZ) GOMASIO AND 160 G (5¾ OZ) TAHINI
Preparation time 5 minutes
Cooking time 5 minutes

Gomasio
250 g (9 oz) white or black sesame seeds
¾ teaspoon fine sea salt

Tahini
125 g (4½ oz) Gomasio
1½ tablespoons sesame oil
2 teaspoons light olive oil

If you prefer to use untoasted sesame seeds, warm the sesame seeds for **5 min/120°C/speed 1**. Add the salt and blend for **20 sec/speed 6**. Transfer to an airtight jar.

To make tahini, blend the gomasio and the oils in the mixer bowl for **30 sec/speed 10**. Scrape down the side of the bowl and blend again.

Both the gomasio and the tahini will keep in an airtight container in the fridge for up to 1 month.

See photograph on pages 40–1.

MAKE AHEAD: FRIDGE
DAIRY-FREE | GLUTEN-FREE | PALEO | VEGAN | VEGETARIAN

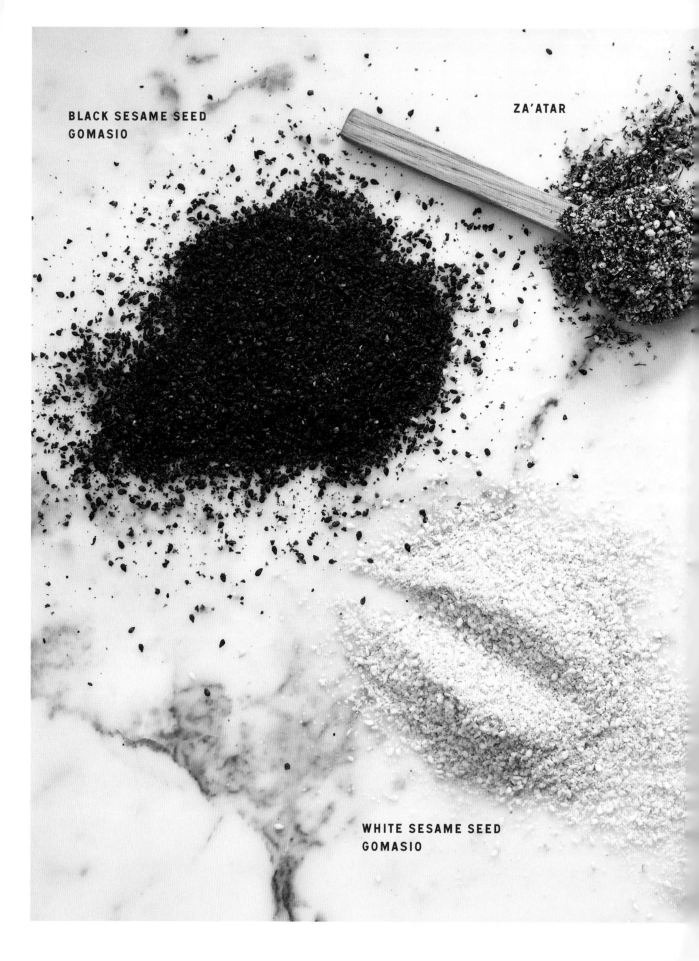

BLACK SESAME SEED
GOMASIO

ZA'ATAR

WHITE SESAME SEED
GOMASIO

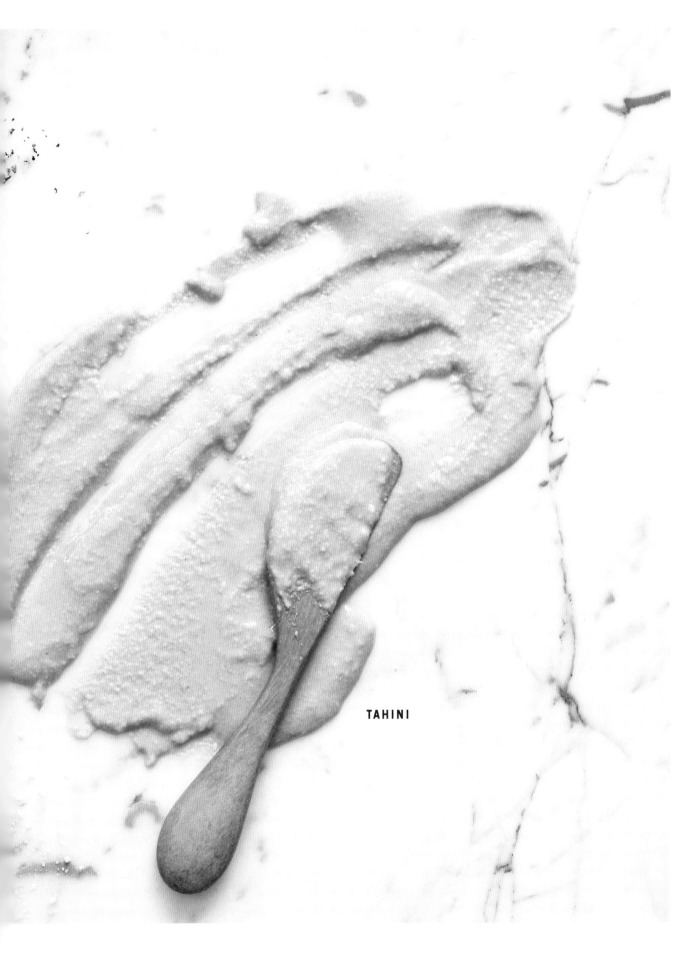

TAHINI

ZA'ATAR

Za'atar is a herb and spice blend used as a dry condiment in Middle Eastern cooking. It can be a little harder to find than other spice blends so I like to make my own. You can find sumac in most supermarkets or in gourmet food stores.

MAKES APPROXIMATELY 125 G (4½ OZ/½ CUP)
Preparation time 5 minutes

2 tablespoons Gomasio (page 39)
2 tablespoons dried thyme
1 tablespoon sumac
2 teaspoons dried oregano
¼ teaspoon fine sea salt

Chop all of the ingredients for **10 sec/speed 8**.

Store in an airtight container in the fridge for up to 2 weeks.

See photograph on page 40.

MAKE AHEAD: FRIDGE
DAIRY-FREE | GLUTEN-FREE | PALEO | VEGAN | VEGETARIAN

ROOT VEG MASH

Steaming vegetables rather than boiling them preserves more of their goodness, as they aren't leaching nutrients into the water during cooking. It also means the vegetables don't have a chance to absorb any water. If using a mixture of vegetables, always put the vegetable that takes longest to cook in the simmering or steaming basket and the quicker-cooking vegetable in the steaming tray.

SERVES 4
Preparation time 10 minutes
Cooking time 15 minutes

800 g (1 lb 12 oz) root vegetables, such as potato, sweet potato, parsnips, swede (rutabaga), or a combination, peeled and cut into 3 cm (1¼ in) pieces
40 g (1½ oz) Butter (page 22) or 2 tablespoons extra virgin olive oil

Add 500 g (1 lb 2 oz) of water to the mixer bowl. Divide the vegetables between the steaming basket and steaming tray, ensuring there are enough clear holes in the basket to allow the steam to pass through to the tray. Attach the steaming basket and tray to the mixer bowl lid.

Cook the vegetables for **15 min/steam mode/ speed 2**, or until tender when pierced with a fork.

Drain the water from the mixer bowl. Add the steamed vegetables, butter or oil and season with sea salt and pepper. Blend for **10 sec/speed 4** then serve.

GLUTEN-FREE | NUT-FREE | PALEO | VEGETARIAN

NUT MILK

When making nut milk, it's best to soak the nuts beforehand. This helps soften them, making them easier to blend so you extract as much of their milk as possible. Soaking is also proven to make them easier to digest and more nutritious because this process unlocks valuable nutrients only released during germination.

Almonds are much harder than macadamias and cashews, so they require longer soaking. You will need to strain the almond milk using a nut-milk bag, but the softer nuts won't require straining.

MAKES 1 LITRE (35 FL OZ/4 CUPS)
Preparation time 5 minutes + soaking time
Soaking time for almonds, pistachios and hazelnuts 8 hours
Soaking time for macadamias and cashews 2 hours

250 g (9 oz/1 cup) mixture of nuts, such as almonds, pistachios, macadamia, cashews and hazelnuts

Place the nuts in a bowl and cover them completely with lukewarm water. Add a good pinch of sea salt, then cover with a tea towel and set aside to soak for the time given above.

Drain the soaked nuts in a sieve and rinse well under plenty of running water. Blend with 1 kg (2 lb 4 oz) of water for **2 min/speed 10**.

Place a nut-milk bag over a large jug or bowl. In batches, pour the milk into the bag, allowing it to strain through – gently squeeze the bag to help the excess milk drain out.

Store the milk in the fridge and use within 2–3 days. Give it a good stir or shake before serving, as it will start to separate over time.

Save any leftover nut meal in the bag for making the Nutty biscuits on page 195. It will keep in the freezer for up to 6 months.

MAKE AHEAD: FRIDGE
DAIRY-FREE | GLUTEN-FREE | PALEO | VEGAN | VEGETARIAN

TIP
One batch of almond nut milk should yield about 100 g (3½ oz) of leftover nut meal. Exactly the right amount to make the Nutty biscuits on page 195.

CHIMICHURRI

Ubiquitous in Argentina and Uruguay, chimichurri dressing turns simple grilled meat into something special. It can also be used as a marinade, salad dressing, or for extra flavour in a steak sandwich. Versatile and delicious.

MAKES 500 ML (17 FL OZ/2 CUPS)
Preparation time 10 minutes

2 vine-ripened tomatoes
1 garlic clove
2 spring onions (scallions), roughly chopped
40 g (1½ oz) flat-leaf (Italian) parsley, including stems, roughly chopped
2 teaspoons dried oregano
½ teaspoon dried chilli flakes
½ teaspoon ground cumin
½ teaspoon sweet paprika
1½ teaspoons raw, white or caster (superfine) sugar
1 teaspoon fine sea salt
4 tablespoons extra virgin olive oil
125 ml (4½ fl oz) red wine vinegar

Using a small sharp knife, score a cross at the top and bottom of each tomato. Place in a heatproof bowl and completely cover with boiling water. Wait for about 30 seconds, or until their skins start to split. Drain and rinse under cold running water to cool, then remove and discard the skins.

Chop all of the ingredients except for the olive oil and vinegar for **5 sec/speed 5**. Scrape down the side of the bowl. Add the oil and vinegar and blend for **4 sec/speed 5**.

Transfer to an airtight container and store in the fridge for up to 5 days.

MAKE AHEAD: FRIDGE

DAIRY-FREE | GLUTEN-FREE | NUT-FREE | VEGAN | VEGETARIAN

HONEY MUSTARD

Making your own jar of mustard is so satisfying, but there is a little waiting time involved. Start this recipe about two weeks before you want to serve it. I use ground turmeric for its colour, but its added goodness is a welcome bonus.

MAKES 300 G (10½ OZ)
Preparation time 5 minutes + standing time

100 g (3½ oz) yellow mustard seeds
125 ml (4 fl oz/½ cup) white wine vinegar
2 teaspoons fine sea salt
3 tablespoons raw honey
½ teaspoon ground turmeric (optional)
2 tablespoons light olive oil

In a bowl, soak the mustard seeds in the vinegar, salt and 150 ml (5 fl oz) of water. Cover with plastic wrap and leave at room temperature for 3 days.

Blend the mustard seed mixture, honey and turmeric, if using, for **20 sec/speed 10**. Scrape down the side of the bowl, including the lid. Repeat the process two more times.

Set the mixer to **20 sec/speed 8**. Slowly add the olive oil through the mixer bowl lid. Continue until the mixture emulsifies.

Transfer the mustard to a sterilised jar (see page 11) with an airtight lid. Seal.

Store in the fridge for up to 1 week before opening and up to 6 months unopened. Once opened, keep refrigerated for up to 1 month.

MAKE AHEAD: FRIDGE

DAIRY-FREE | GLUTEN-FREE | NUT-FREE | PALEO | VEGETARIAN

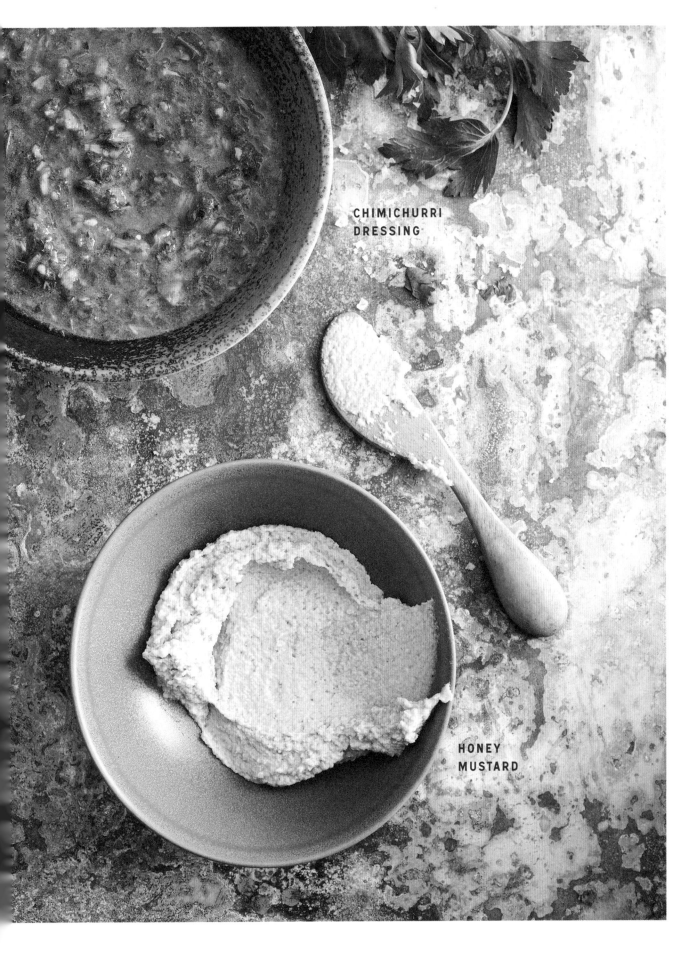

CHIMICHURRI
DRESSING

HONEY
MUSTARD

MY NOT-TOO-SWEET CHILLI SAUCE

I'm not a huge fan of the sickly sweet sweet chilli sauces available in supermarkets. I much prefer giving my family a homemade version. If you like your chilli sauce with a bit of a kick, throw a couple of bird's eye chillies in the mix to make up the total chilli weight. Since rice syrup isn't as sweet as palm or raw sugar, I start off with 1 tablespoon of fish sauce first, then taste and add as I go. It's always better to start with a smaller amount of an ingredient to help balance the flavours than it is to overdo it. If using palm sugar, you can add it at the beginning when chopping up the chillies.

MAKES APPROXIMATELY 250 ML (9 FL OZ/1 CUP)

Preparation time 10 minutes
Cooking time 30 minutes

50 g (1¾ oz) long red chillies, stems removed, roughly chopped
1 garlic clove
1 lemongrass stem, tough outer stems discarded, roughly chopped
110 g (3¾ oz/½ cup) rice syrup, grated palm sugar (jaggery) or raw sugar
125 ml (4 fl oz/½ cup) rice wine vinegar
1–1½ tablespoons fish sauce, to taste

Chop the chillies, garlic and lemongrass for **10 sec/speed 7**. Scrape down the side of the bowl.

Add the rice syrup, vinegar and 2 tablespoons water. Attach the simmering basket, instead of the measuring cup, to the mixer bowl lid. Cook for **30 min/100°C/speed 2**. Add the fish sauce for the last minute of cooking.

Pour the hot sauce into warm sterilised jars (see page 11) with airtight lids and seal. Turn the jars upside down on a heatproof surface and leave to cool.

Store the sauce in a cool, dark place for up to 6 months. Once opened, keep refrigerated for up to 1 month.

See photograph on page 49.

MAKE AHEAD: PANTRY | FRIDGE
DAIRY-FREE | GLUTEN-FREE | NUT-FREE

MAYONNAISE

Mass-produced mayos are often packed with nasties and a long list of ingredients you've never heard of. Fresh is always best, that way you know exactly what's going in it.

For me personally, aioli (or garlic mayonnaise) is just that little bit more exciting, not to mention a little better for you.

MAKES APPROXIMATELY 300 G (10½ OZ)

Preparation time 5 minutes

1 garlic clove (optional, use if making aioli)
1 tablespoon lemon juice (add 2 additional teaspoons, if you want a lemon mayonnaise)
1 egg
2 teaspoons Honey mustard (page 44) or dijon mustard
½ teaspoon fine sea salt
250 ml (9 fl oz/1 cup) grapeseed or light olive oil

If you're going to make aioli, chop the garlic for **3 sec/speed 7**. Scrape down the side of the bowl.

Add the lemon juice, egg, mustard and salt. Blend for **2 min/speed 4**, while very slowly pouring the oil through the mixer bowl lid. Continue until the mixture emulsifies and turns into a thick mayonnaise.

Store the aioli or mayonnaise in an airtight container in the fridge for up to 1 week.

See photograph on page 48.

MAKE AHEAD: FRIDGE
DAIRY-FREE | GLUTEN-FREE | NUT-FREE | PALEO | VEGETARIAN

RANCH DRESSING

Like mayonnaise, ranch dressings that are commercially produced are often full of ingredients that are less than fresh. If you have some aioli to hand, it couldn't be easier to make your own. Once you do, you won't look back.

MAKES 250 ML (9 FL OZ/1 CUP)

Preparation time 5 minutes

125 ml (4 fl oz/½ cup) Buttermilk (page 22)
125 ml (4 fl oz/½ cup) aioli (see left)

Blend the buttermilk and aioli for **30 sec/ speed 4**.

Use the dressing immediately, or store it in an airtight container for up to 3 days. Give it a good shake or stir before use.

See photograph on page 49.

MAKE AHEAD: FRIDGE
GLUTEN-FREE | NUT-FREE | PALEO | VEGETARIAN

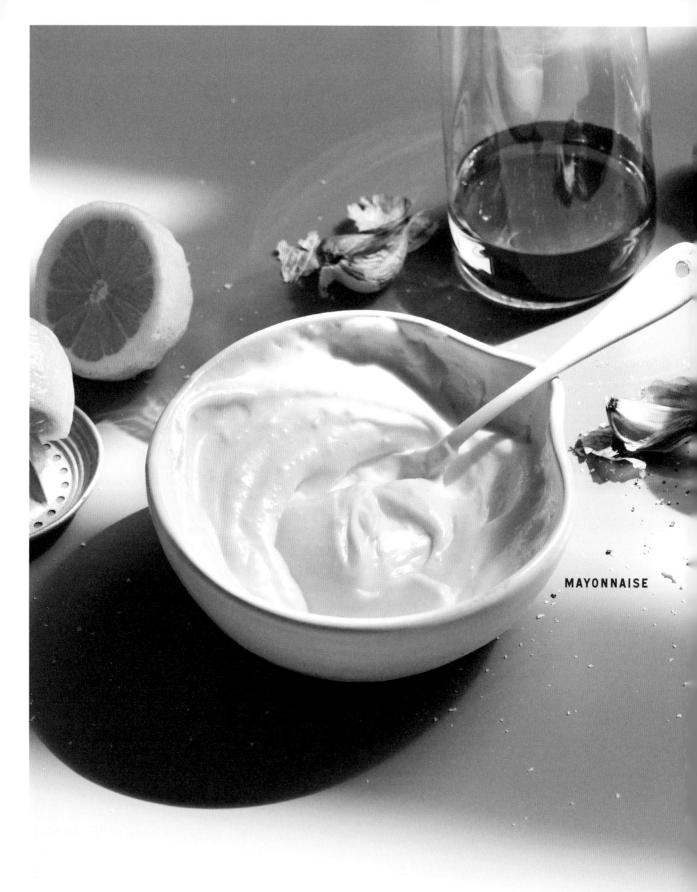

MAYONNAISE

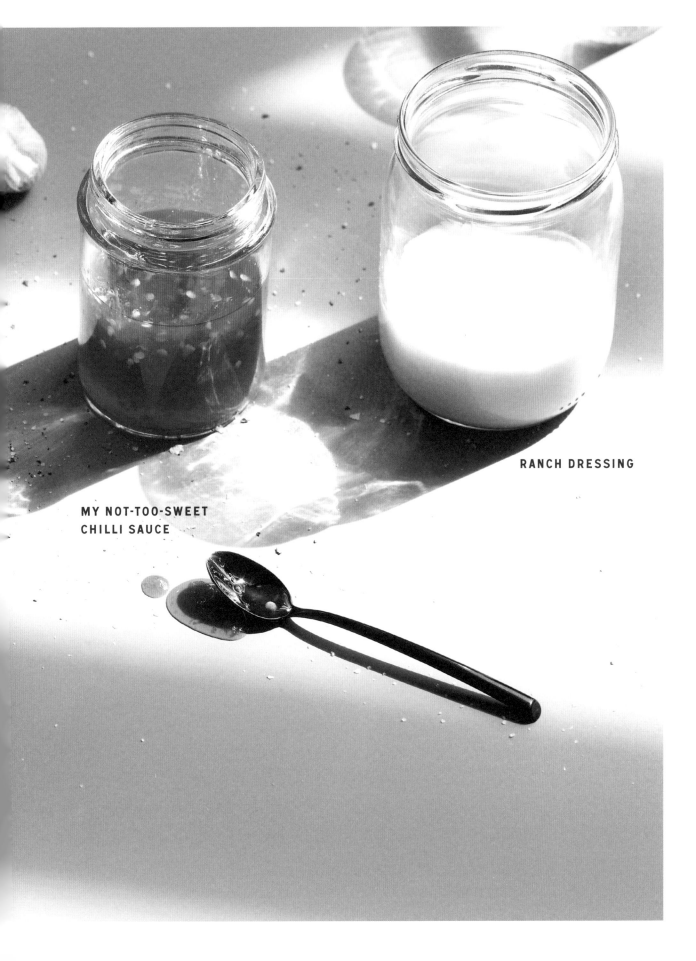

RANCH DRESSING

MY NOT-TOO-SWEET
CHILLI SAUCE

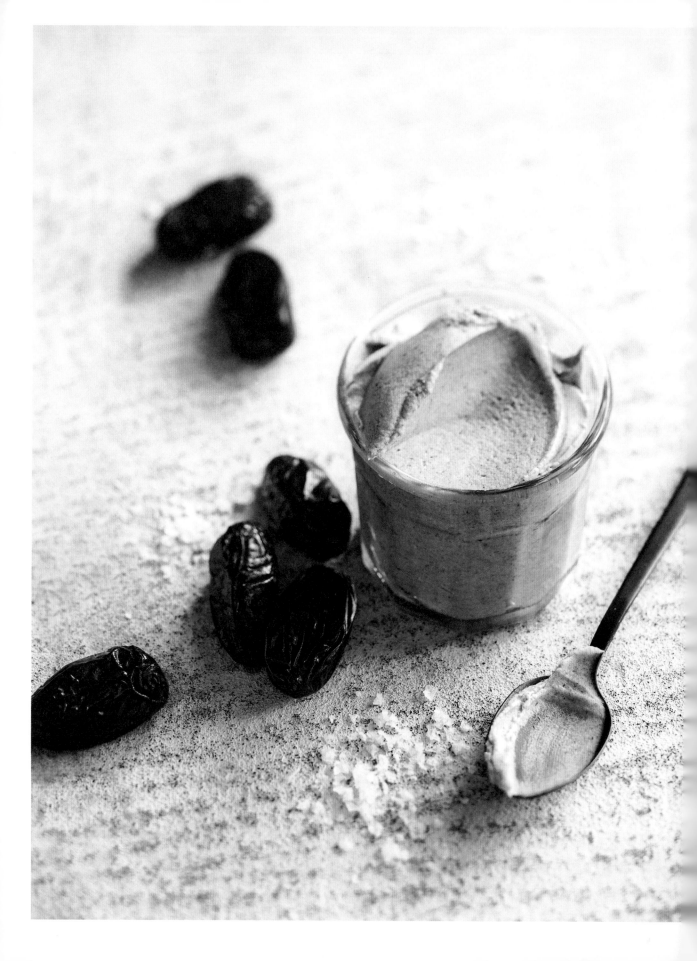

VEGAN SALTED CARAMEL SAUCE

This vegan caramel sauce is a great alternative to traditional caramels, which use sugar, butter and cream. And the good news is that it's just as delicious. How much salt you'll need will depend on the sweetness of the dates, so start with a little and add to your taste. This keeps well but once it's been in the fridge it really firms up. To bring it back, gently heat it up in the microwave until it is warm and has a pouring consistency. It's delicious drizzled over so many things, from fresh fruit to puddings.

MAKES APPROXIMATELY 375 ML (13 FL OZ/1½ CUPS)

Preparation time 5 minutes
Cooking time 15 minutes

200 g (7 oz/1¼ cups) fresh dates, pitted
270 ml (9½ fl oz) coconut cream
¾ teaspoon fine sea salt

Blend all of the ingredients for **15 sec/speed 8**. Scrape down the side of the bowl, then repeat the process. Cook for **15 min/100°C/speed 2**. Blend for **15 sec/speed 8** until nice and smooth.

Store the caramel sauce in an airtight jar or container in the fridge for up to 1 week.

MAKE AHEAD: FRIDGE
DAIRY-FREE | GLUTEN-FREE | NUT-FREE | VEGAN | VEGETARIAN

SUPER SOUPS

CHICKEN AND BLACK BEAN TORTILLA SOUP

Tortilla soup is a traditional Mexican dish that is typically made with chicken. Here, I've added black beans to make it an even heartier number that works well with less chicken. If pickled jalapeños are too spicy for your family, just leave them out or use less than I've suggested.

SERVES 4

Preparation time 10 minutes
Cooking time 25 minutes

1 red onion, peeled and quartered
1–2 tablespoons pickled jalapeños
1 teaspoon smoked paprika
1 teaspoon ground cumin
1 tablespoon neutral oil, such as rice bran or grapeseed oil, plus extra to drizzle
1 litre (35 fl oz/4 cups) Chicken stock (page 31)
400 g (14 oz) Naked pasta sauce (page 14) or tinned chopped tomatoes
100 g (3½ oz) dried black beans, cooked, or 400 g (14 oz) tinned black beans, rinsed and drained
4 corn tortillas, halved, cut into 1 cm (½ in) strips
250 g (9 oz) chicken breast stir-fry strips
finely grated zest and juice of 1 lime
15 g (½ oz/½ cup) coriander (cilantro), stems and leaves roughly chopped
crumbled feta or goat's cheese, to serve

Preheat the oven to 180°C (350°F). Chop the onion, jalapeños, spices and oil for **5 sec/speed 5**. Scrape down the side of the bowl. Cook for **3 min/120°C/speed 1**. Add the stock, pasta sauce and beans and season well with salt. Cook for **15 min/90°C/speed 1**.

Meanwhile, place the tortilla strips on a baking tray, lightly drizzle with oil and season with salt. Arrange in a single layer. Bake in the oven for 12 minutes, or until golden and crisp. Remove and set aside.

Add the chicken, lime juice, zest and half the coriander to the soup. Cook for **5 min/90°C/reverse stir/speed 1**, or until the chicken is cooked through.

Serve with crispy tortilla strips, cheese and remaining coriander.

MAKE AHEAD: FREEZER
GLUTEN-FREE | NUT-FREE | PALEO

TIP

This freezes well for up to 3 months, but if that's your plan, don't add the chicken or make the tortilla strips until after you've defrosted and reheated the soup.

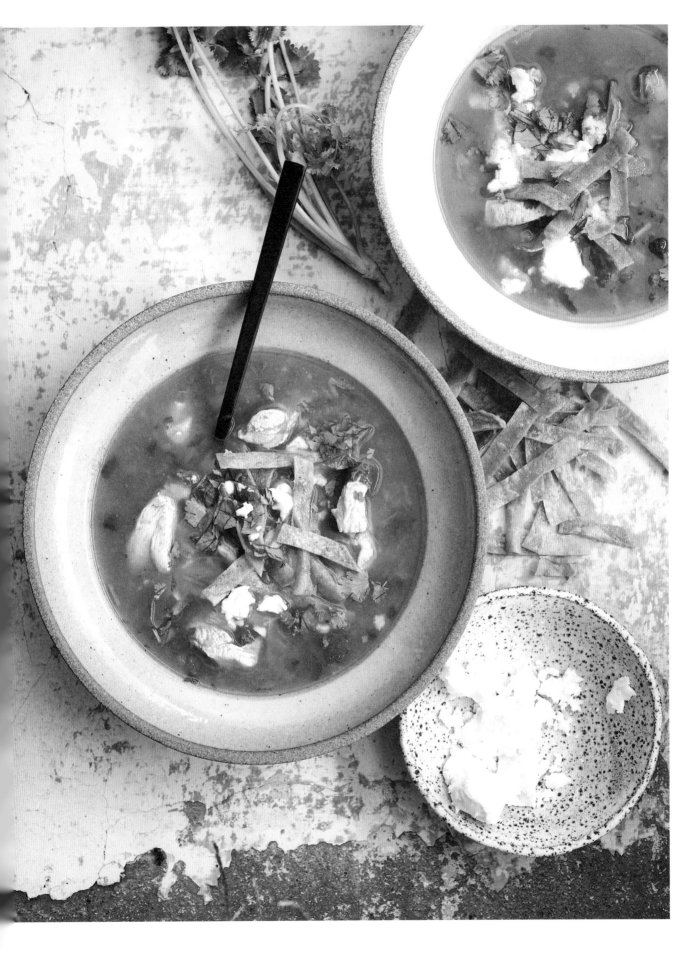

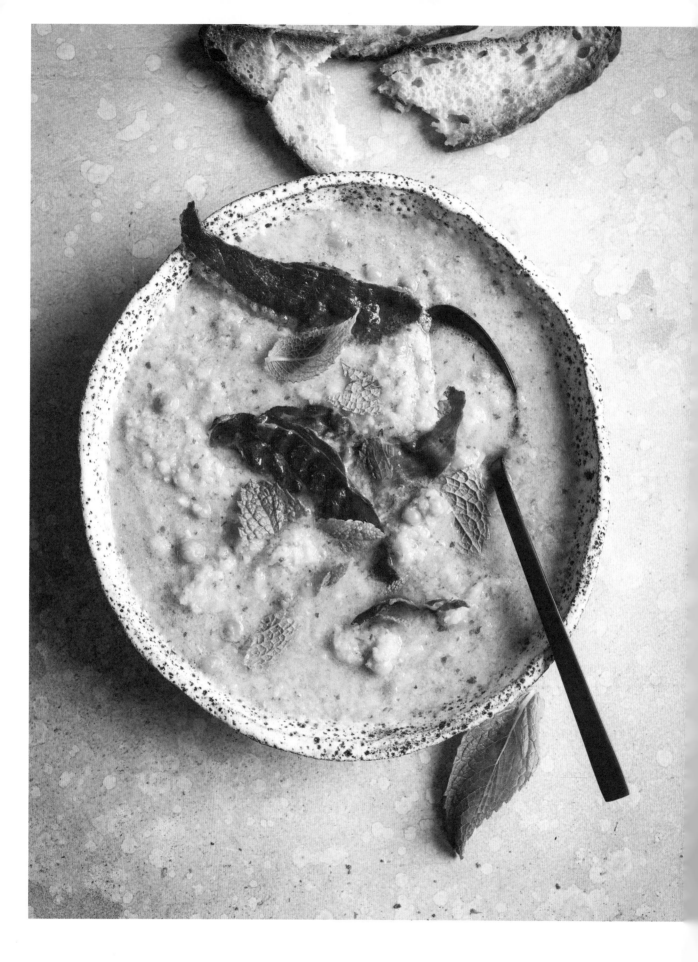

THE NEW PEA AND 'HAM' SOUP

Introducing my lighter, fresher, quicker AND healthier take on a traditional classic, pea and ham soup. How many more reasons do you need to give this version a try? The soup base can be frozen for up to 6 months in an airtight container and then finished off just before serving. Top the soup with feta instead of prosciutto and use vegetable stock (page 32) instead of chicken stock to make it a vegetarian number.

SERVES 4

Preparation time 10 minutes
Cooking time 10 minutes

1 leek, white part only, roughly chopped
2 garlic cloves
250 g (9 oz) starchy potatoes, peeled and roughly chopped
2 tablespoons thyme leaves
1 tablespoon extra virgin olive oil, plus extra to serve
1 litre (35 fl oz/4 cups) Chicken stock (page 31)
2 zucchini (courgettes), thinly sliced
500 g (1 lb 2 oz) frozen peas
1 large handful mint leaves
100 g (3½ oz) prosciutto slices (you can also use pancetta or bacon)
No-work 'sourdough' bread, to serve (page 23)

Chop the leek, garlic, potato and thyme for **5 sec/speed 5**. Scrape down the side of the bowl. Add the oil and season with sea salt and pepper. Cook for **3 min/120°C/speed 1**.

Add the chicken stock, zucchini, two-thirds of the peas and half of the mint. Cook for **5 min/100°C/speed 1**.

Meanwhile, heat a large frying pan over medium heat. Cook the prosciutto for a minute or two on each side until golden and crisp. Remove and drain on paper towel.

Blend the soup for **30 sec/speed 6**, or until smooth. Add the remaining peas and cook for **2–3 min/100°C/speed 1** until heated through. Season to taste with salt and pepper.

Serve the soup topped with the crispy prosciutto, reserved mint, a drizzle of extra virgin olive oil and some crusty bread.

MAKE AHEAD: FREEZER

DAIRY-FREE | NUT-FREE

LEMON, CHICKEN AND RICE SOUP

This is the best healing chicken soup you will find. The combination of turmeric, garlic and lemon together with lean chicken and vitamin-rich greens will have you feeling good in no time. You need to serve this soup immediately, otherwise the rice absorbs the liquid rather quickly. It's best to start off with less lemon juice and add to taste.

SERVES 4

Preparation time 5 minutes
Cooking time 15 minutes

2 garlic cloves
2.5 cm (1 in) piece of turmeric, peeled or 1 teaspoon ground turmeric
2–3 tablespoons lemon juice
150 g (5½ oz) long-grain rice, rinsed and drained
1.25 litres (44 fl oz/5 cups) Chicken stock (page 31)
150 g (5½ oz) baby spinach leaves
400 g (14 oz) chicken breast stir-fry strips
1 handful coriander (cilantro), leaves and stems finely chopped

Chop the garlic and turmeric for **5 sec/speed 7**. Scrape down the side of the bowl.

Add the lemon juice, rice and chicken stock. Cook for **12 min/95°C/reverse stir/speed 1**. Add the spinach and chicken. Cook for **4 min/95°C/reverse stir/speed 1**, or until the chicken is cooked through. Season to taste with sea salt and pepper.

Scatter over the coriander then serve.

DAIRY-FREE | GLUTEN-FREE | NUT-FREE

COCONUT AND LIME FISH SOUP

You can't go wrong with a creamy coconut-based soup, especially when you add in the persuasive fragrance of kaffir lime leaves. This is a good option for both warmer and cooler months, and it can be easily adapted by using a combination of prawns and fish, or by mixing up the veggies. Add the fish sauce and lime juice to taste, starting with a little and working up to more until the flavours are just right.

SERVES 4

Preparation time 10 minutes
Cooking time 15 minutes

2 spring onions (scallions), whites and greens roughly chopped
1–2 long green chillies, seeds removed, roughly chopped
2 celery stalks, roughly chopped
1 x 400 ml (14 fl oz) tin coconut cream
750 ml (26 fl oz/3 cups) Seafood stock (page 33)
1 lemongrass stem, cut into 10 cm (4 in) lengths, lightly pounded
    with a rolling pin
6 kaffir lime leaves, 5 scrunched up and 1 finely shredded, to serve
500 g (1 lb 2 oz) boneless, skinless firm white fish fillets,
    such as ling, diced into 2.5 cm (1 in) pieces
2 zucchini (courgettes), halved lengthways and thinly sliced
100 g (3½ oz) sugar snap peas, trimmed
2–3 tablespoons fish sauce
2–3 tablespoons lime juice

Chop the spring onions, green chilli and celery for **10 sec/speed 10**. Scrape down the side of the bowl and repeat the process.

Add the coconut cream and blend for **10 sec/speed 10**. Add the stock, lemongrass and the five scrunched-up lime leaves. Cook for **10 min/90°C/speed 1**.

Add the fish, zucchini, sugar snap peas, fish sauce and lime juice. Cook for **5 min/90°C/speed 1**, or until the fish is cooked and the vegetables are tender.

Serve the soup with the shredded kaffir lime leaf scattered on top.

DAIRY-FREE | GLUTEN-FREE | NUT-FREE | PALEO

SUPERFOOD CHICKEN CONGEE

The silver lining whenever I stayed home sick from school was that Mum would make a large bowl of congee. Typically, congee is eaten for breakfast, but I enjoy it any time of day. Using super grains makes this comforting dish even healthier and gives it a lower GI.

SERVES 4

Preparation time 10 minutes
Cooking time 30 minutes

3 garlic cloves
3 spring onions (scallions), white parts reserved, green parts thinly sliced
25 g (1 oz) ginger, peeled and roughly chopped
1 large handful coriander (cilantro), sprigs picked, stems reserved
1 litre (35 fl oz/4 cups) Chicken stock (page 31)
200 g (7 oz/1 cup) tricolour quinoa, soaked in water for at least 30 minutes, drained and rinsed
2 teaspoons chia seeds (optional)
2 x 150 g (5½ oz) skinless chicken breasts
optional toppings: sesame oil, tamari, chopped toasted almonds, white pepper

Chop the garlic, white parts of the spring onions, ginger and coriander stems for **5 sec/speed 6**. Scrape down the side of the bowl.

Add the chicken stock, quinoa and chia seeds, if using. Place the chicken into the simmering basket and season well with salt and pepper, then insert the basket into the mixer bowl. Cook for **15 min/90°C/speed 2**, or until the chicken is cooked through. Carefully remove the simmering basket and chicken and set aside to rest for 10 minutes. Continue to cook the soup for **15 min/100°C/speed 2,** or until the mixture resembles porridge.

After the chicken has rested, use two forks to shred it into large pieces. Serve the congee with the chicken, coriander sprigs and spring onion greens scattered on top, and any additional toppings you like.

DAIRY-FREE | GLUTEN-FREE | PALEO

TIP

When it comes to flavours, this is such a versatile soup. Use minced pork and prawns instead of chicken, or seafood (if you do this, use a seafood stock for the base rather than a chicken stock). It can easily satisfy vegetarians too by using vegetable stock rather than chicken, adding extra veg and topping with a soft-boiled egg.

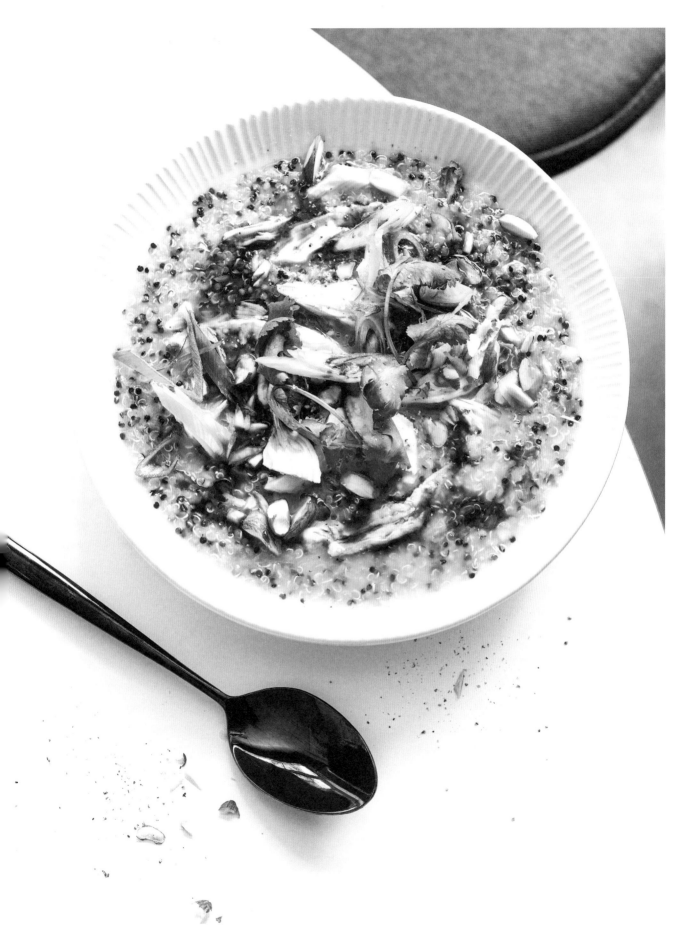

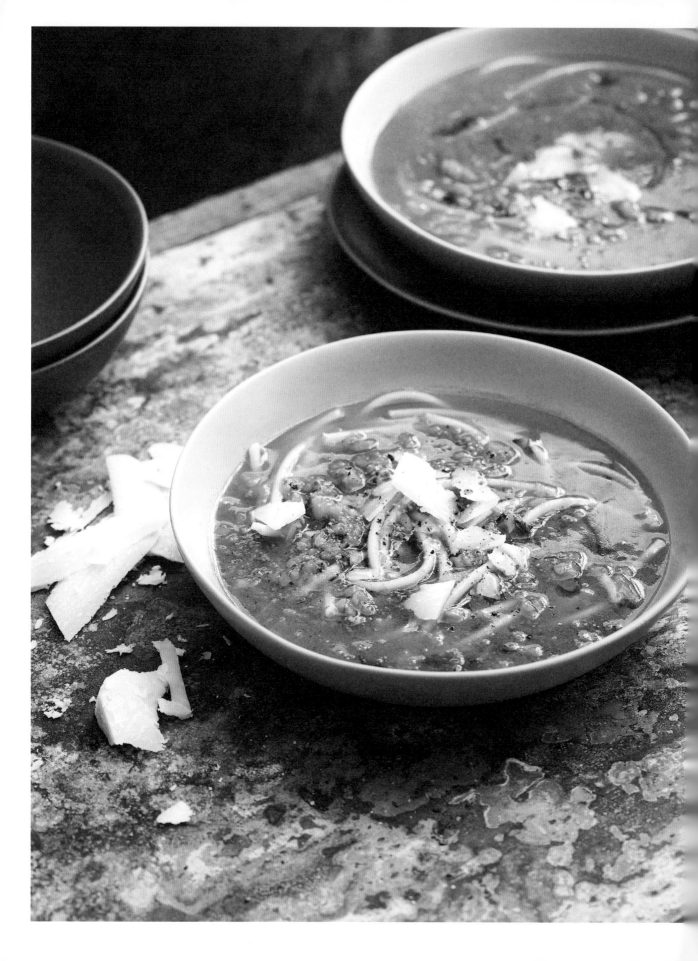

BEEF RAGU PASTA AND TOMATO SOUP

The idea of a spag bol soup may be difficult to get your head around, but trust me, your family won't be able to get the spoons in their mouths fast enough! The base is really all about the homemade pasta sauce and chicken stock. It's definitely worth taking those extra steps for this twist on a family favourite. Keep in mind that it's best to serve the soup immediately as the pasta soaks up the liquid rather quickly.

SERVES 4

Preparation time 10 minutes
Cooking time 30 minutes

2 carrots, peeled and roughly chopped
2 celery stalks, roughly chopped
1 tablespoon extra virgin olive oil, plus extra to serve
400 g (14 oz) minced (ground) beef
3 tablespoons fresh oregano leaves
800 g (1 lb 12 oz) Naked pasta sauce (page 14) or tinned chopped tomatoes
500 ml (17 fl oz/2 cups) Chicken or Vegetable stock
   (pages 31 and 32), or water
200 g (7 oz) bucatini pasta, broken into thirds
shaved parmesan cheese, to serve

Chop the carrots and celery for **4 sec/speed 5**. Scrape down the side of the bowl. Add the oil and cook for **3 min/120°C/speed 1**.

Add the minced beef and oregano and season with sea salt and pepper. Cook for **5 min/120°C/speed 1**.

Add the pasta sauce and stock and cook for **10 min/100°C/speed 1**. Remove the measuring cup, so steam can escape, then carefully add the pasta through the hole in the lid. Return the measuring cup and cook for **10 min/100°C/speed 1**, or until the pasta is al dente.

Serve the soup immediately topped with parmesan and a drizzle of extra virgin olive oil.

MAKE AHEAD: FREEZE
NUT-FREE

TIP

You can double the soup (leaving the pasta out) and freeze it in batches for up to 3 months, adding the pasta and the cheese after reheating. You could also cook the pasta separately.

SUNSET SOUP

Step aside pumpkin soup, here's an even better way of getting a whole bunch of nutrient-dense vegetables into your family. This soup reminds me of a warm sunset, hence the name. You can easily add a little more or a little less of the orange vegetables, as long as you end up with the same total veg weight as below, that's fine. This freezes well in an airtight container for up to 6 months.

SERVES 4

Preparation time 10 minutes
Cooking time 20 minutes

1 leek, white part only, roughly chopped
2 garlic cloves
1 carrot, peeled and roughly chopped
1 tablespoon extra virgin olive oil, plus extra to serve
250 g (9 oz) peeled pumpkin (winter squash), cut into 3 cm (1¼ in) pieces
400 g (14 oz) sweet potato, peeled and cut into 3 cm (1¼ in) pieces
750 ml (26 fl oz/3 cups) Vegetable stock (page 32)
2 teaspoons fine sea salt
Labne (page 27) and Za'atar (page 42) or dukkah, to serve

Chop the leek, garlic and carrot for **4 sec/speed 5**. Scrape down the side of the bowl. Add the oil and cook for **3 min/120°C/speed 1**.

Add the pumpkin, sweet potato, stock and salt. Cook for **15 min/95°C/ speed 2** or until the vegetables are tender. Blend for **30 sec/speed 5**, then increase to **speed 8** for a further **15 seconds**, or until the soup is smooth.

Top with a spoonful of labne, a drizzle of extra virgin olive oil and a pinch of za'atar, then serve.

MAKE AHEAD: FREEZE
GLUTEN-FREE | PALEO | VEGETARIAN

POTATO, LEEK AND CORN SOUP

Just the simple step of adding corn takes this family favourite to a whole new level. Kids and big kids will love it just the same. You can store it in an airtight container for up to 6 months.

SERVES 4

Preparation time 10 minutes
Cooking time 25 minutes

2 leeks, white part only, roughly chopped
30 g (1 oz) Butter (page 22)
2 corn cobs, kernels removed
500 g (1 lb 2 oz) starchy potatoes, peeled and roughly chopped
750 ml (26 fl oz/3 cups) Vegetable stock (page 32)
chopped chives (optional), to serve
extra virgin olive oil (optional), to serve

Chop the leeks for **10 sec/speed 5**. Scrape down the side of the bowl. Add the butter and cook for **3 min/120°C/speed 1**.

Add half the corn kernels to the steaming basket, then add the rest to the mixer bowl with the potatoes and stock. Season well with salt and pepper. Attach the steaming basket, instead of the measuring cup, to the mixer bowl lid. Cook for **20 min/ 100°C/speed 2**.

Blend for **30 sec/speed 5**, then increase to **speed 8** for a further **30 seconds**. Add more water if you'd like a thinner consistency.

Add the steamed corn to the soup and season to taste with sea salt and pepper. Mix for **20 sec/speed 2**.

Serve the soup with chives and a drizzle of extra virgin olive, if you like.

MAKE AHEAD: FREEZE
GLUTEN-FREE | NUT-FREE | PALEO | VEGETARIAN

FRENCH ONION SOUP

Using chicken stock instead of beef makes this soup a little lighter than the original version. I prefer using white cheeses for this, but feel free to use any combination of cheeses you enjoy the most. You can freeze the soup in an airtight container in the freezer for up to 6 months.

SERVES 4
Preparation time 10 minutes
Cooking time 35 minutes

4 red onions, peeled and quartered
2 garlic cloves
2 tablespoons thyme leaves
40 g (1½ oz) Butter (page 22)
1.5 litres (52 fl oz/6 cups) Chicken stock (page 31)
1 tablespoon Honey mustard (page 44) or dijon mustard
1 tablespoon apple cider vinegar
200 g (7 oz) mixture of feta cheese, chopped haloumi and goat's cheese
4 slices of No-work 'sourdough' (page 23)
extra virgin olive oil, to drizzle

Chop the onions, garlic and thyme for **4 sec/speed 4**. Scrape down the side of the bowl. Add the butter and cook for **15 min/120°C/speed 1**.

Add the stock, mustard and vinegar and cook for **20 min/95°C/speed 1**. Season to taste with salt and pepper.

Meanwhile, crumble or break up the cheeses and combine them in a small bowl.

Preheat the oven grill (broiler) to high. Drizzle both sides of the bread with oil and place on a large baking tray. Grill for 1–2 minutes on one side and until lightly golden on the other, then remove.

Spread the cheese mixture on the lightly toasted side of each slice of bread. Divide the soup between serving bowls, place those on an oven tray, then set a piece of toast over each bowl. Place under the grill for 3 minutes, or until the cheese is lightly golden and warmed through then serve immediately.

MAKE AHEAD: FREEZE
NUT-FREE

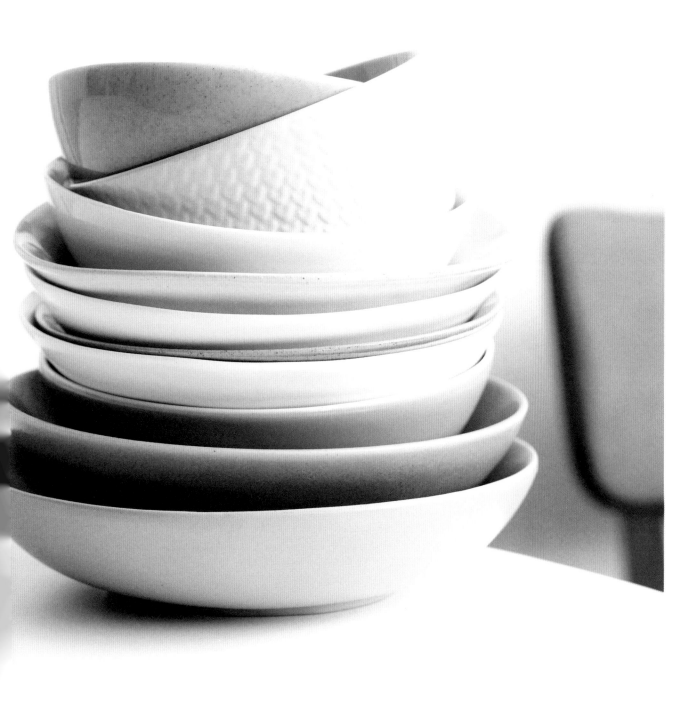

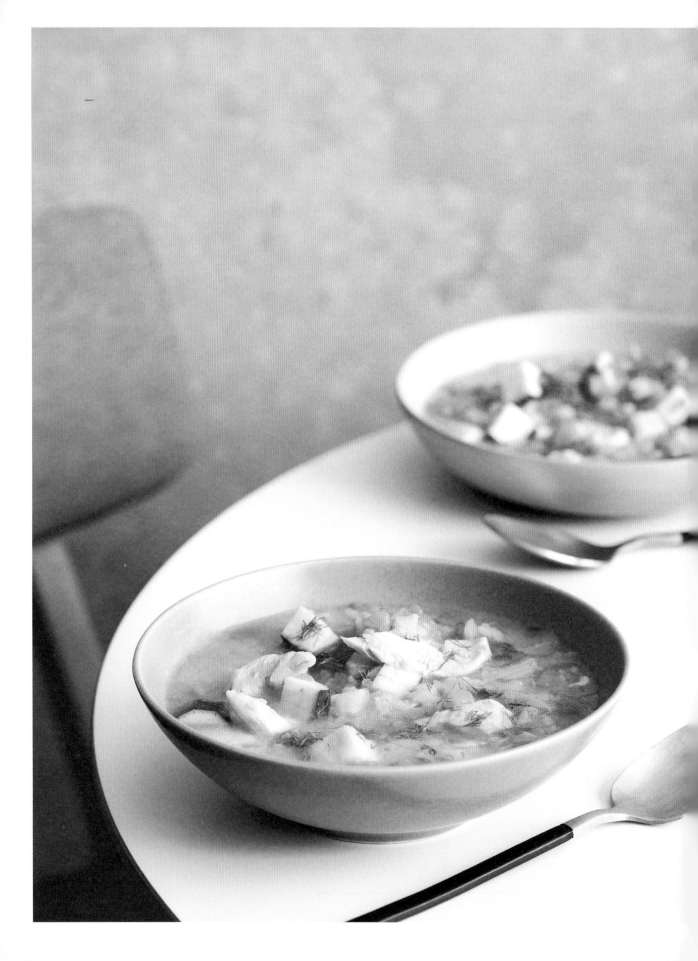

CHICKEN, VEGETABLE AND BARLEY SOUP

This is my healthier take on chicken noodle soup. I like to add pearl barley, a nutty grain, in place of pasta. I also use whole toasted coriander or fennel seeds – they add a special little pop of something to a lot of soups and are a pleasant surprise in any mouthful.

SERVES 4

Preparation time 10 minutes
Cooking time 45 minutes

2 garlic cloves
2 carrots, peeled and roughly chopped
2 celery stalks, roughly chopped
1 fennel bulb, roughly chopped, fronds reserved and finely chopped
1 teaspoon coriander or fennel seeds, toasted
4 fresh or dried bay leaves
1 tablespoon extra virgin olive oil, plus extra to drizzle
1 litre (35 fl oz/4 cups) Chicken stock (page 31)
75 g (2¾ oz/⅓ cup) pearl barley
1 zucchini (courgette), cut into 1.5 cm (⅝ in) pieces
400 g (14 oz) chicken breast stir-fry strips

In two batches, chop the garlic, carrots, celery and fennel for **2 sec/speed 5**. Scrape down the side of the bowl and return the first batch of vegetables to the mixer bowl.

Add the coriander seeds, bay leaves and oil. Cook for **3 min/120°C/speed 1**.

Add the chicken stock and pearl barley. Cook for **35 min/95°C/speed 1**. Add the zucchini and chicken and cook for a further **5 min/90°C/reverse stir/speed 1**, or until the chicken is cooked through. Season to taste with salt and pepper.

Serve the soup with some chopped fennel fronds scattered on top and a drizzle of extra virgin olive oil.

MAKE AHEAD: FREEZER
DAIRY-FREE | GLUTEN-FREE | NUT-FREE

TIP

You can make this soup in advance and freeze it in an airtight container without the chicken for up to 6 months, then thaw the soup out in the fridge. Add the chicken once the soup is hot and continue cooking from that point in the method.

SMOKY SEAFOOD SOUP

This is my smokier take on the classic French seafood stew bouillabaisse. A seafood soup fit for kings and queens (and their families).

SERVES 4
Preparation time 10 minutes
Cooking time 25 minutes

a pinch of saffron threads (optional)
1 fennel bulb, roughly chopped, fronds reserved and finely chopped, to serve
2 celery stalks, roughly chopped
1 red onion, peeled and roughly chopped
1 tablespoon extra virgin olive oil, plus extra to serve
1 tablespoon smoked paprika
400 g (14 oz) Naked pasta sauce (page 14) or tinned chopped tomatoes
750 ml (26 fl oz/3 cups) Seafood stock (page 33)
500 g (1 lb 2 oz) cleaned and debearded mussels
200 g (7 oz) raw peeled green prawns (shrimp)
400 g (14 oz) boneless, skinless fish fillets, such as salmon or
    firm white fish, cut into 4 cm (1½ in) pieces
slices of No-work 'sourdough' (page 23), chargrilled, to serve
aioli (page 47), to serve

Soak the saffron, if using, in 1 tablespoon of warm water. Meanwhile, chop the fennel for **5 sec/speed 5**. Transfer to a bowl and set aside. Add the celery and onion and chop for **5 sec/speed 5**. Return the fennel to the mixer bowl and scrape down the side of the bowl.

Add the oil and smoked paprika and season with salt and pepper. Cook for **5 min/120°C/speed 1**.

Add the pasta sauce, stock and the saffron and its soaking liquid. Place the mussels in the steaming basket and attach that to the mixer bowl lid. Cook for **15 min/steam mode/speed 2**. Put the prawns and fish in the simmering basket and carefully insert it into the mixer bowl. Reattach the steaming basket with the mussels to the mixer bowl lid.

Cook for **5 min/steam mode/speed 1**, or until the mussels have popped open and the fish and prawns are cooked through. Divide the soup, then the seafood evenly between the serving bowls. Top with fennel fronds then serve with bread, aioli and a drizzle of oil.

DAIRY-FREE | NUT-FREE

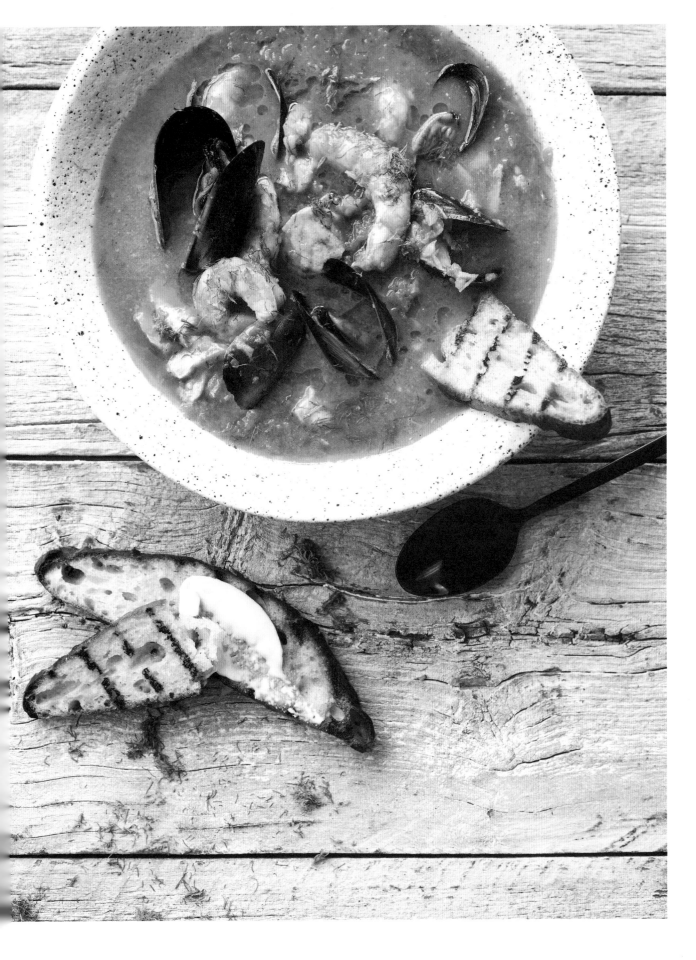

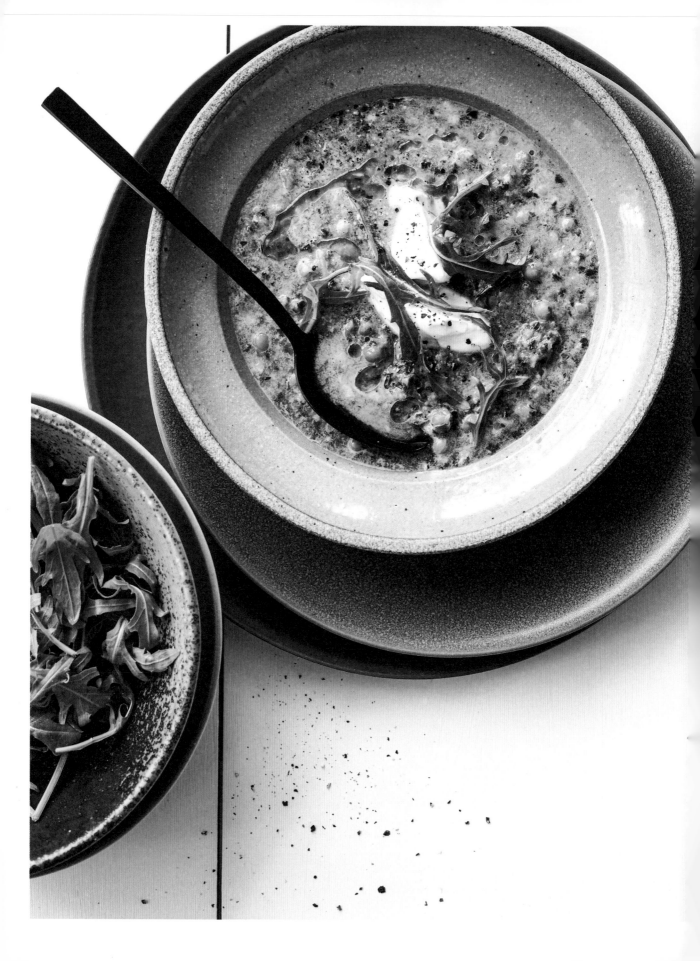

GREEN GODDESS SOUP

I love this soup, and so does everyone I've ever served it to. Not only will it make you feel superhuman, it also treats your body like a temple. Because every ingredient is alkalising, it is one of the best soups in this book to make if you're after something to keep your family going and growing. It also happens to be really delicious. You can store this in the freezer in an airtight container for up to 6 months.

SERVES 4

Preparation time 5 minutes
Cooking time 10 minutes

3 garlic cloves
4 zucchini (courgettes), roughly chopped
2 tablespoons extra virgin olive oil, plus extra to drizzle
200 g (7 oz) baby spinach leaves
1 litre (35 fl oz/4 cups) unsweetened coconut water
50 g (1¾ oz) rocket (arugula) leaves
500 g (1 lb 2 oz) frozen peas
100 g (3½ oz) goat's Labne (page 27), Homemade goat's yoghurt
   (page 26) or goat's cheese

Chop the garlic and zucchini for **2 sec/speed 5**. Scrape down the side of the bowl. Add the oil and cook for **3 min/120°C/speed 1**.

Add the spinach, coconut water, most of the rocket and half of the peas. Season with salt and pepper. Cook for **5 min/100°C/speed 2**.

Blend for **30 sec/speed 6**. Scrape down the side of the bowl. Add the remaining peas and cook for **3 min/100°C/speed 1**, or until hot. Season to taste with salt and pepper.

Serve the soup topped with a few rocket leaves, a drizzle of extra virgin olive oil and a dollop of goat's labne.

MAKE AHEAD: FREEZE
GLUTEN-FREE | NUT-FREE | PALEO | VEGETARIAN

MISO CHICKEN RAMEN

Some ramen stocks take up to 24 hours to prepare, but this one can be made in next to no time. You can use fresh or dried ramen noodles and serve this with different cuts of chicken.

SERVES 4

Preparation time 10 minutes + standing time
Cooking time 20 minutes

4 dried shiitake mushrooms
500 ml (17 fl oz/2 cups) boiling water
2 carrots, peeled and roughly chopped
1 leek, white part only, roughly chopped
2 garlic cloves
4 cm (1½ in) piece of ginger, peeled and roughly chopped
1 litre (35 fl oz/4 cups) Chicken stock (page 31)
1 tablespoon sesame oil, plus extra to serve
2 tablespoons tamari (gluten-free soy sauce)
2 tablespoons mirin
1 tablespoon honey
100 g (3½ oz) white miso paste
500 g (1 lb 2 oz) skinless chicken thigh fillets, trimmed and cut into thirds
350 g (12 oz) dried ramen noodles
1 spring onion (scallion), thinly sliced, to serve
2 boiled eggs, halved
Gomasio (page 39), to serve

Place the mushrooms in a heatproof jug or bowl and pour in the boiling water. Cover the jug with a plate and leave to soak for 10 minutes. Meanwhile, chop the carrots, leek, garlic and ginger for **3 sec/speed 5**. Scrape down the side of the bowl.

Remove and discard the stems from the mushrooms before adding to the mixer bowl with their soaking liquid, the chicken stock and sesame oil. Cook for **10 min/100°C/speed 2**.

Add the tamari, mirin, honey and miso paste to the mixer bowl. Place the chicken in the simmering basket and carefully insert into the mixer bowl. Cook for **10 min/95°C/speed 2**, or until the chicken is cooked through.

Meanwhile, cook the noodles according to the packet instructions. Serve the soup topped with the sliced chicken, spring onion, halved eggs and gomasio.

DAIRY-FREE

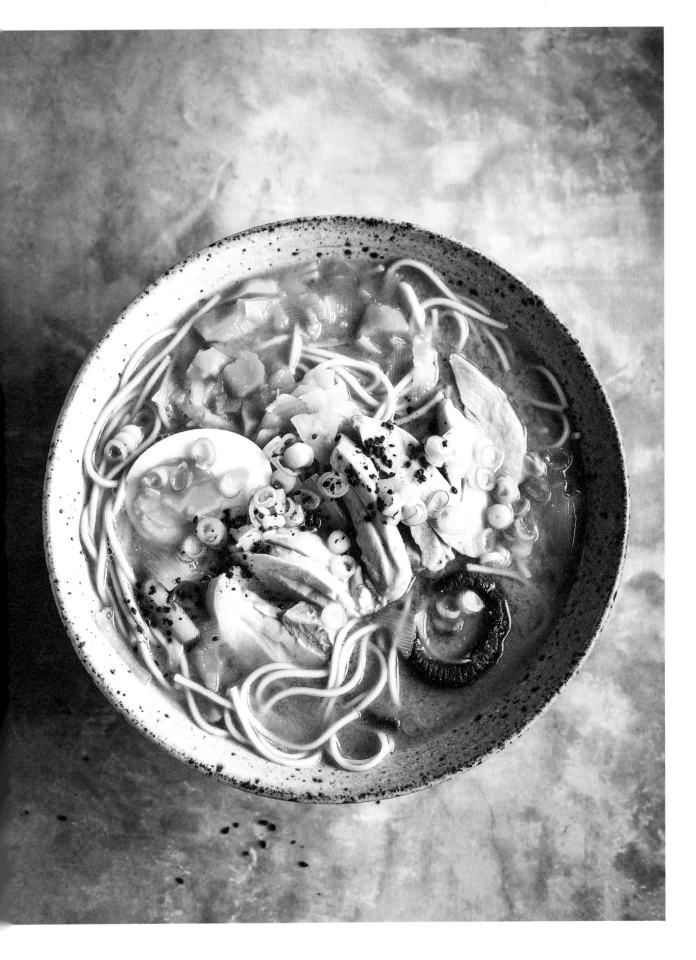

CHILLED AVOCADO SOUP WITH CRUNCHY CORN AND PEPITAS

This chilled soup has all the personality and kick of a good guacamole, and who doesn't love guacamole? This cool little number is a great way to trick the kids into eating a really nutritious soup, especially in the warmer months when a hot soup is the last thing anyone wants to eat. Avocados got a bad rap for a while when healthy fats were out of favour, but thankfully that time is over and we are free to devour these beauties to our heart's content. Best to keep all of the ingredients for this refrigerated, that way it will be chilled and ready to serve as soon as you've made it.

SERVES 4

Preparation time 15 minutes

1 corn cob, kernels removed
4 tablespoons lime juice
2 ripe avocados, stones removed, peeled
3 Lebanese (short) cucumbers, peeled, roughly chopped
2 spring onions (scallions), roughly chopped
250 ml (9 fl oz/1 cup) unsweetened coconut water
2 tablespoons extra virgin olive oil
260 g (9¼ oz/1 cup) Homemade goat's yoghurt (page 26), plus extra to serve
1 small handful coriander (cilantro), leaves picked, stems roughly chopped
2 teaspoons fine sea salt
toasted pepitas (pumpkin seeds), to serve

Combine the corn kernels and lime juice in a bowl and set aside for at least 10 minutes to lightly pickle or 'cook' the corn.

Put the avocado, cucumber, spring onion, coconut water, oil, yoghurt, coriander stems and salt in the mixer bowl. Pour the corn into a sieve set over the mixer bowl and let the lime juice collect in the bowl. Blend for **20 sec/speed 8**.

Serve the soup topped with a dollop of goat's yoghurt, then scatter over some corn kernels, pepitas and coriander leaves to finish.

See photograph on page 78.

GLUTEN-FREE | PALEO | VEGETARIAN

WATERMELON GAZPACHO

It doesn't get much easier or refreshing than this cold soup. It's the perfect way to cool down in the heat of the sun. Hello, summer!

SERVES 4–6

Preparation time 10 minutes

2 Lebanese (short) cucumbers, peeled and halved
1 kg (2 lb 4 oz) seedless watermelon flesh, roughly chopped
2 vine-ripened tomatoes, quartered
½ small red onion
3 tablespoons red wine vinegar
mint leaves, to serve
extra virgin olive oil, to serve

Cut a good-sized chunk off one of the cucumber halves. Finely chop that chunk and set aside.

Add all of the remaining ingredients to the mixer bowl and season with salt and pepper. Blend for **20 sec/speed 9**.

Serve topped with the finely chopped cucumber, a few mint leaves and a drizzle of extra virgin olive oil.

See photograph on page 79.

DAIRY-FREE | GLUTEN-FREE | NUT-FREE | PALEO | VEGAN | VEGETARIAN

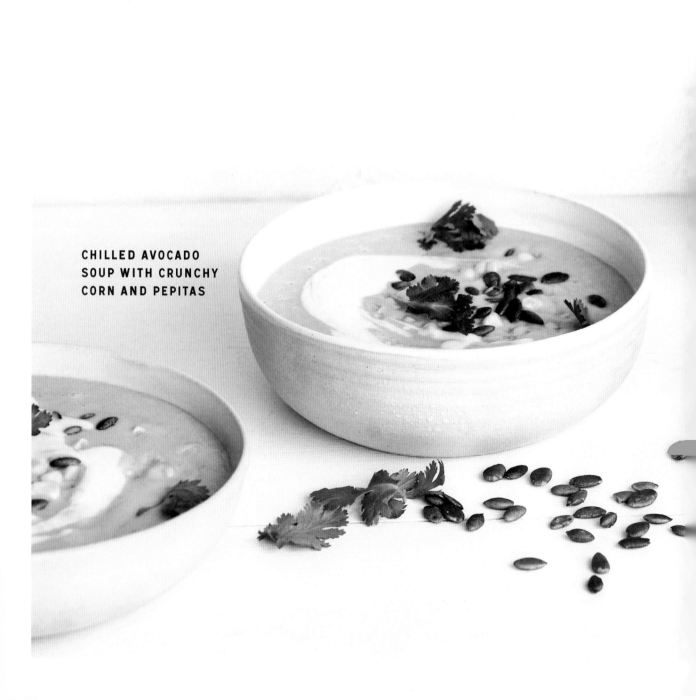

CHILLED AVOCADO
SOUP WITH CRUNCHY
CORN AND PEPITAS

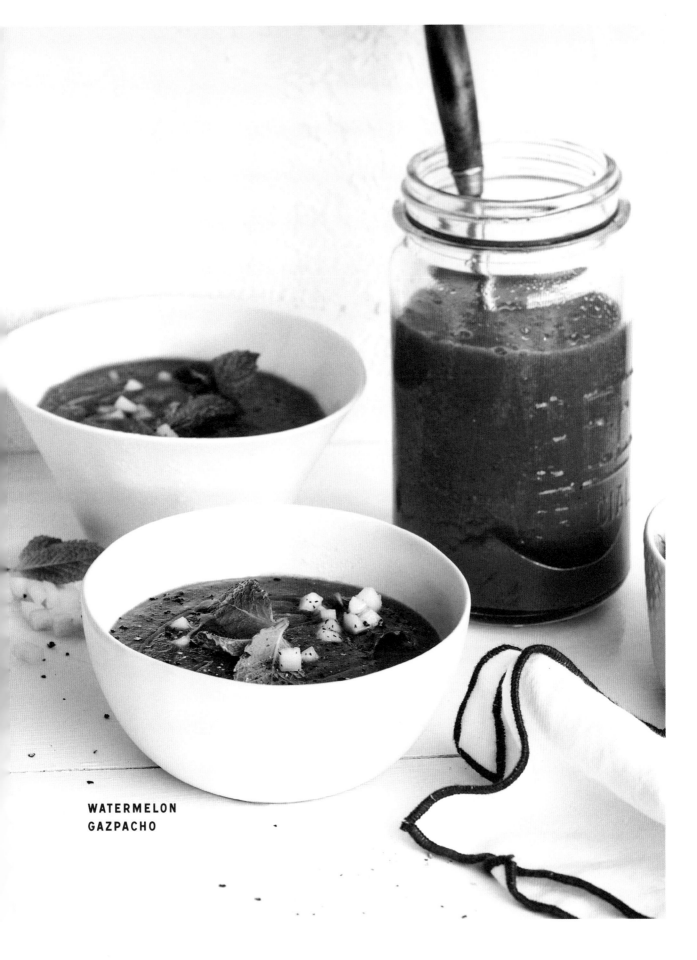

WATERMELON
GAZPACHO

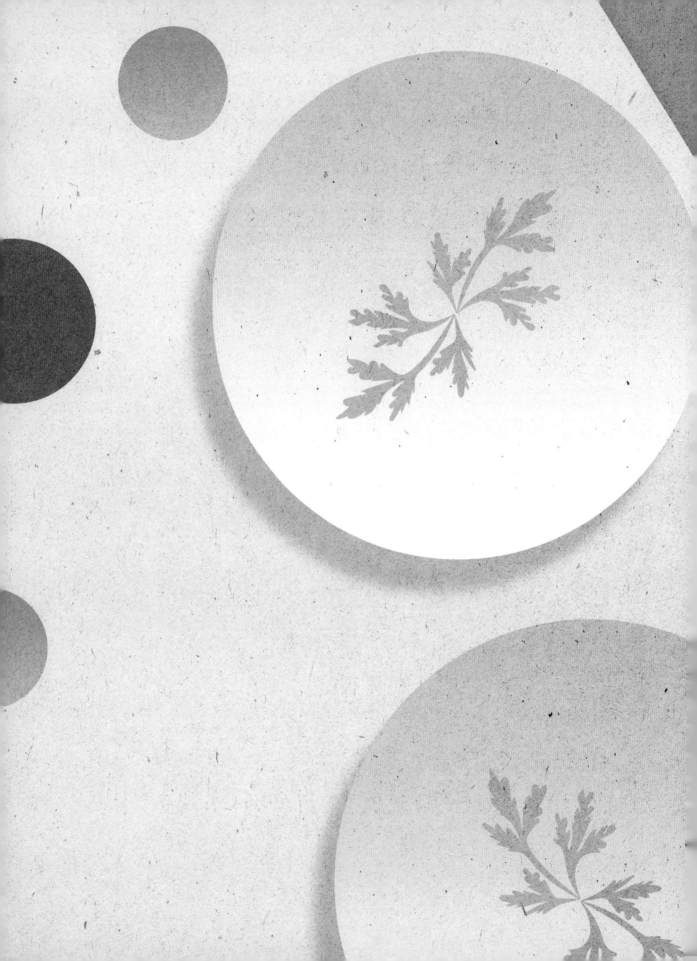

WEEKNIGHT WONDERS

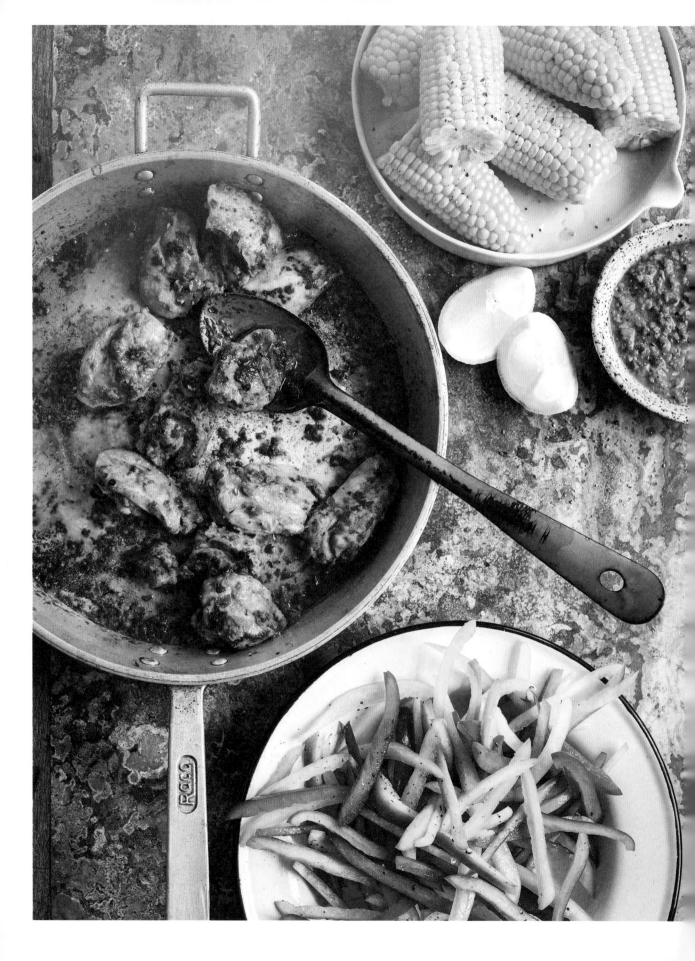

PIRI PIRI CHICKEN

If you're trying to introduce spice to the younger members of your family, this piri piri recipe is a good place to start, being pretty low on the heat radar. It's also great on the barbecue. The sauce can be made in advance and stored in the fridge for up to 5 days, or frozen for up to 6 months. You can also marinate the chicken then freeze it.

SERVES 4

Preparation time 10 minutes + standing time
Cooking time 10 minutes

2 lemons, 1 zested and juiced,
   1 cut into wedges, to serve
6 long red chillies, seeds removed,
   roughly chopped
6 garlic cloves
2 teaspoons smoked paprika
3 tablespoons fresh oregano leaves
4 tablespoons olive oil

1 teaspoon fine sea salt
600 g (1 lb 5 oz) skinless chicken
   thigh fillets, trimmed, cut into thirds
4 corn cobs, husks removed, halved
   crossways
3 capsicums (peppers), red, green
   and yellow, stems and seeds
   removed, cut into thin strips

Blend the lemon juice and zest, chilli, garlic, paprika, oregano, oil and salt for **8 sec/speed 6**.

Add the chicken to a bowl with 4 tablespoons of the marinade and mix until well combined. Set aside to marinate for at least 15 minutes. Reserve the remaining marinade for serving.

Pour 500 g (1 lb 2 oz) of water into the mixer bowl. Divide the corn between the simmering basket and steaming basket. Attach the steaming basket, instead of the measuring cup, to the mixer bowl lid. Cook for **10 min/steam mode/speed 2**, or until cooked.

Meanwhile, heat a large non-stick frying pan over medium heat. Add the chicken and partially cover with a lid. Cook the chicken for 4 minutes each side, or until charred and cooked through. Remove the chicken from the pan and set aside to rest for 5 minutes. Meanwhile, combine the sliced capsicum in a bowl.

Serve the chicken with the corn, capsicum, remaining sauce and lemon wedges.

MAKE AHEAD: FRIDGE | FREEZER
DAIRY-FREE | GLUTEN-FREE | NUT-FREE | PALEO | LOW-CARB

CHEAT'S HAINANESE CHICKEN RICE

Make a broth, cook rice, *and* steam chicken and vegetables all at the same time for this cheat's version of Singapore's national dish. Your thermo deserves a round of applause!

SERVES 4

Preparation time 20 minutes + standing time
Cooking time 25 minutes

6 spring onions (scallions), roughly chopped
60 g (2¼ oz) ginger, peeled and roughly chopped
4 garlic cloves
2 tablespoons sesame oil
1 litre (35 fl oz/4 cups) Chicken stock (page 31)
1¼ teaspoons fine sea salt
freshly ground white pepper
300 g (10½ oz) jasmine rice, rinsed
2 x 250 g (9 oz) chicken breasts
500 g (1 lb 2 oz) Chinese broccoli, trimmed, thinly sliced
1½ tablespoons rice wine vinegar
2 teaspoons raw sugar
kecap manis, to serve (see Note)

Chop the spring onion, ginger and garlic with 1 tablespoon of the sesame oil for **5 sec/speed 6**. Scrape down the side of the bowl and repeat this process two more times. Transfer half of the mixture to a bowl. Add the stock, 1 teaspoon of the salt and some white pepper, if you like, to the mixer bowl, then add the rice to the simmering basket.

Season the chicken then place it in the steaming basket. Attach the steaming basket to the mixer bowl lid. Cook for **12 min/100°C/speed 4**. Meanwhile, place the broccoli on the steaming tray.

Add the remaining sesame oil, the vinegar, sugar, remaining salt and 2 teaspoons of water to the bowl with the spring onion mixture, and stir until the sugar dissolves. After the rice has been cooking for 12 minutes, carefully remove the simmering basket and place it in a large bowl. Cover the bowl with a plate and set aside until ready to serve.

Attach the steaming basket and tray to the mixer bowl lid. Cook for a further **10 min/steam mode/speed 2**, or until the chicken is cooked and the broccoli is tender. Remove the steaming basket and tray from the mixer bowl and set aside for 5 minutes to rest then slice the chicken.

Serve the chicken with the rice, broccoli, broth, sauce and kecap manis.

DAIRY-FREE | GLUTEN-FREE | PALEO

NOTE
Kecap manis is a dark, sweet syrupy Indonesian soy sauce, available in Asian supermarkets.

JERK CHICKEN WITH COCONUT AND CORN RICE

Jerk recipes usually include some of the hottest chillies on earth, but I've really toned down the heat so that everyone can enjoy it. Green chillies are generally mild, but feel free to use less if you prefer. This is a great one for the barbecue.

SERVES 4

Preparation time 15 minutes + standing time
Cooking time 20 minutes

1 teaspoon black peppercorns
4 spring onions (scallions), roughly chopped
4 garlic cloves
2 jalapeño chillies or 4 long green chillies, roughly chopped (remove seeds to lower the heat factor)
2 tablespoons thyme leaves
2 tablespoons ground allspice
2 cm (¾ in) piece of ginger, peeled

2 teaspoons ground cinnamon
2 teaspoons maple syrup
2 limes, 1 juiced, 1 cut into wedges
3 tablespoons coconut oil
2 teaspoons fine sea salt
500 g (1 lb 2 oz) skinless chicken thigh fillets, trimmed and halved
2 corn cobs, kernels removed
300 g (10½ oz) long-grain rice, rinsed

Mill the peppercorns for **20 sec/speed 10**. Add the spring onion, garlic, chillies, herbs and spices, maple syrup, lime juice, 2 tablespoons of the coconut oil and the salt. Blend for **30 sec**, starting at **speed 1** and slowly increasing to **speed 6**.

Transfer the marinade to a bowl with the chicken and mix until well coated. Set aside for at least 10 minutes (overnight is best) to marinate.

Add 1 kg (2 lb 4 oz) of water to the mixer bowl. Combine the corn and rice in the simmering basket. Insert the simmering basket into the mixer bowl. Cook for **18 min/100°C/speed 4** until the rice is tender. Season the rice with salt and stir in the remaining coconut oil to combine. Cover, then leave to stand for at least 5 minutes.

Meanwhile, heat a large frying pan over medium heat. Add the chicken, partially cover with a lid and cook for 8–10 minutes, turning every minute, until charred and cooked through. Remove and set aside to rest for 5 minutes before serving with the rice and lime wedges.

MAKE AHEAD: FREEZE
DAIRY-FREE | GLUTEN-FREE | NUT-FREE | PALEO

THAI-STYLE BROWN RICE FISH CAKES

Fish cakes are one of those family favourites that are hard to refuse. The great thing about these ones is that they are a meal in one: fish, rice, vegetables and wonderfully fragrant flavours in one little package! I like using brown basmati rice because it's quick, and also a good source of essential nutrients.

SERVES 4

Preparation time 15 minutes + standing time
Cooking time 30 minutes

225 g (8 oz) brown basmati rice, rinsed and drained
3 teaspoons chia seeds (optional)
8 kaffir lime leaves, stems removed
600 g (1 lb 5 oz) boneless, skinless firm white fish fillets, roughly chopped
1 egg, plus 1 egg white, lightly beaten
75 g (2¾ oz) red curry paste
3 teaspoons rice syrup or sugar
250 g (9 oz) green beans, trimmed and thinly sliced
coconut oil, for frying
mixed salad leaves, to serve
My not-too-sweet chilli sauce (page 46), to serve

Preheat the oven to 100°C (200°F). Add 1 kg (2 lb 4 oz) of water to the mixer bowl. Place the rice into the simmering basket and insert into the mixer bowl. Cook for **15 min/100°C/speed 4** until the rice is tender. Carefully remove and set aside to cool. Meanwhile, soak the chia seeds, if using, in 2 tablespoons of water.

Chop the kaffir lime leaves for **5 sec/speed 7**. Add the fish and chop for **3 sec/speed 4**. Scrape down the side of the bowl. Add the soaked chia, rice, egg and egg white, curry paste, rice syrup and salt. Blend for **5 sec/speed 5**. Scrape down the side of the bowl. Add the beans and mix for **10 sec/speed 3**.

Using slightly damp hands, shape the mixture into 12 fish cakes about 2.5 cm (1 in) thick. Heat the oil in a large frying pan over medium heat then cook the fish cakes in batches for 2–3 minutes each side, or until golden and cooked through. Keep them warm in the oven as you go, then serve right away with salad leaves and sweet chilli sauce.

GLUTEN-FREE | DAIRY-FREE | NUT-FREE

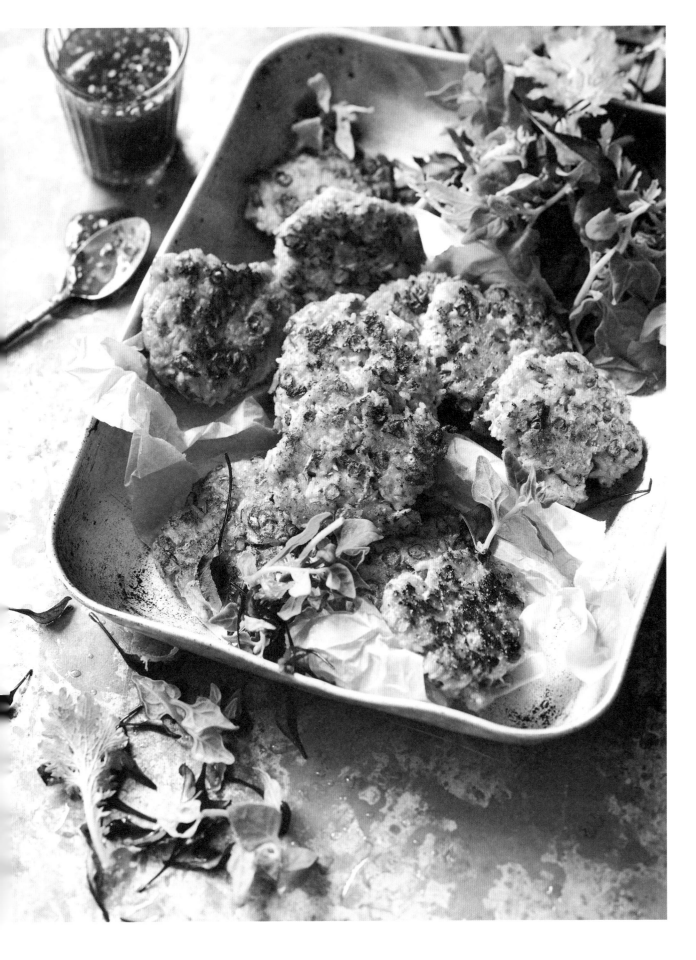

MISO AND BLACK SESAME CHICKEN WITH APPLE AND CUCUMBER KIMCHI

You can use white or black gomasio for this recipe, or even whole sesame seeds if you prefer. Personally, I find using black gomasio for this recipe that little bit more fun; wait until you get it to the table! The apple kimchi is definitely another great thing to try if you're looking to encourage the family to give something new a go.

SERVES 4

Preparation time 25 minutes
Cooking time 10 minutes

Apple and cucumber kimchi
40 g (1½ oz) ginger, peeled
1 garlic clove
1–2 long red chillies, seeds removed, roughly chopped (optional)
3 Lebanese (short) cucumbers, halved, seeds scooped out, roughly chopped
2 green apples, peeled, quartered and cored
1 large carrot, peeled and roughly chopped
1 teaspoon fine sea salt
100 g (3½ oz) sweet potato noodles (see Note) or bean thread noodles, broken up
2 tablespoons tamari (gluten-free soy sauce)
1 tablespoon rice syrup, maple syrup or sugar
1 handful chives, cut into 2 cm (¾ in) lengths

Miso and black sesame chicken
2 tablespoons white miso paste
1½ tablespoons sesame oil
500 g (1 lb 2 oz) chicken tenderloins, trimmed
100 g (3½ oz) black or white Gomasio (page 39)

Preheat the oven to 220°C (425°F) and line a baking tray with baking paper.

Chop the ginger, garlic and chilli, if using, for **3 sec/speed 8**. Scrape down the side of the bowl. Add the cucumbers and chop for **2 sec/speed 4**. Transfer the mixture to a serving bowl.

Chop the apples and carrot for **2 sec/speed 5**. Transfer to the serving bowl with the cucumbers, add the salt and mix until very well combined.

Set aside for at least 10 minutes to lightly pickle, then drain through a fine-mesh sieve and return to the serving bowl.

Meanwhile, combine the miso paste with 1 tablespoon of the sesame oil in a large, wide-based bowl or dish. Add the chicken and mix until well coated. Add the gomasio to a plate or shallow dish. Roll the chicken in the gomasio until well coated then place on the lined tray in a single layer and bake for 8 minutes, or until cooked through. Remove from the oven and set aside to rest for 4 minutes.

Meanwhile, bring 1 kg (2 lb 4 oz) of water to the boil for **5 min/100°C/ speed 2**. Add the noodles and cook them according to the packet instructions on **reverse stir/speed 2**. Drain and rinse under cold running water to cool completely. Cut the noodles into shorter lengths with scissors.

Combine the tamari, rice syrup and the remaining sesame oil in a bowl, then add this sauce mixture to the kimchi, along with the chives and noodles. Mix until well combined.

Slice the chicken, then serve with the kimchi.

See photograph on pages 90–1.

See photograph on pages 90–1.

DAIRY-FREE | GLUTEN-FREE

NOTE

You should be able to find Korean sweet potato noodles in an Asian supermarket. Alternatively, you can use bean thread or rice vermicelli noodles as a substitute.

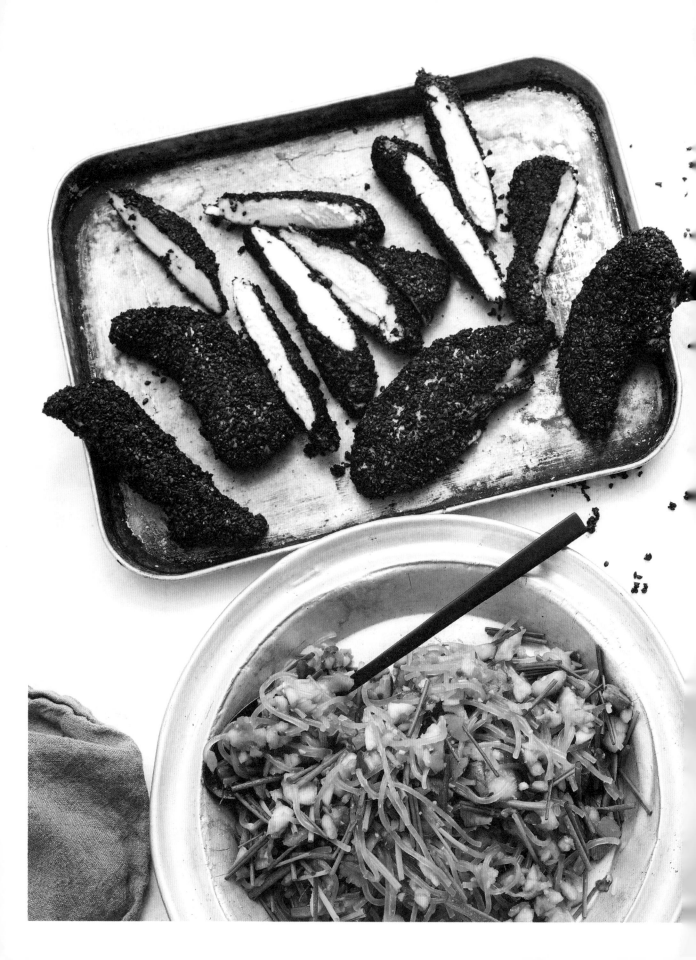

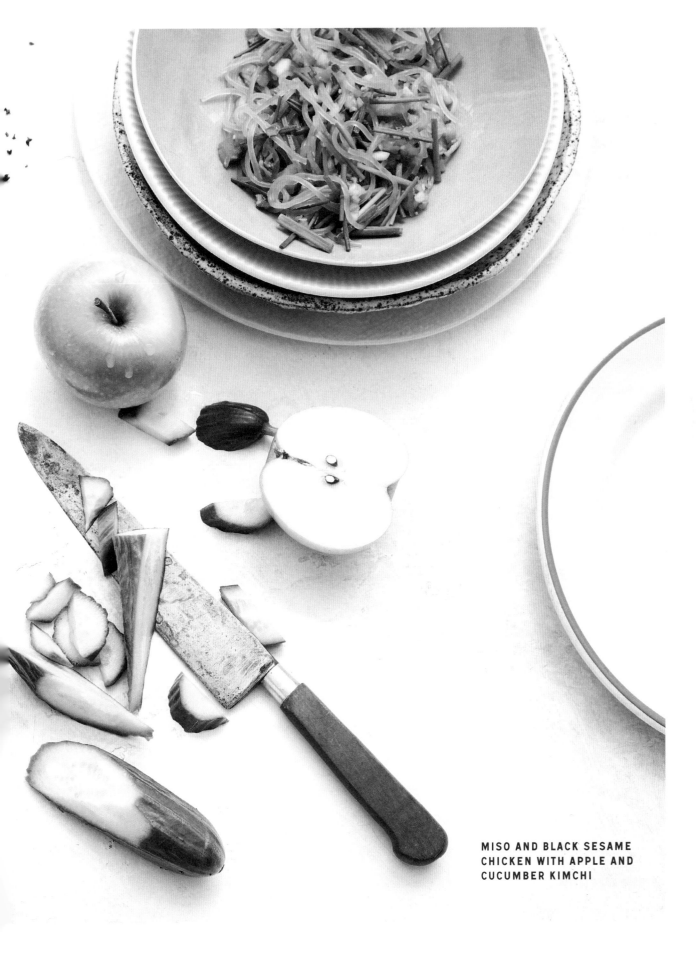

MISO AND BLACK SESAME
CHICKEN WITH APPLE AND
CUCUMBER KIMCHI

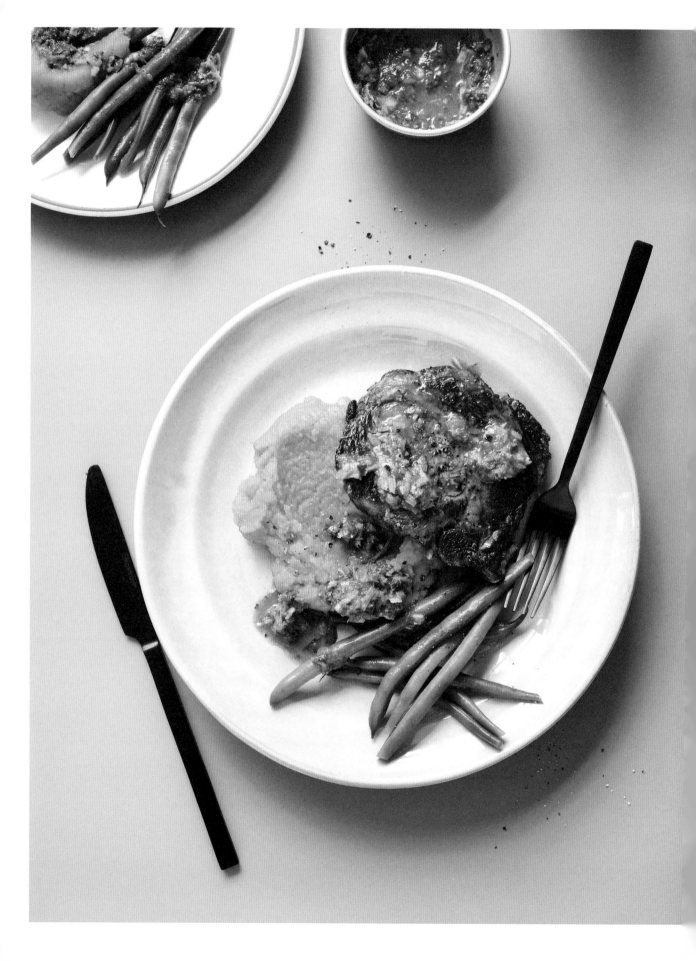

BEEF WITH CHIMICHURRI AND SWEET POTATO MASH

Always a crowd pleaser, it doesn't get any easier to win the family over on a weeknight than with this dish. The chimichurri dressing can be made ahead of time so all you need to do to bring things together is let your mixer prepare the mash while you cook the steaks to perfection. The flavours here work equally well with lamb steaks.

SERVES 4

Preparation time 15 minutes
Cooking time 25 minutes

1 quantity sweet potato mash (follow method on page 42), to serve
500 g (1 lb 2 oz) green beans, topped
1 tablespoon olive oil
4 x 150 g (5½ oz) beef steaks, such as Scotch fillet
Chimichurri (page 44), to serve

Make the sweet potato mash, then transfer the mash to a bowl and cover to keep warm. Clean the mixer bowl then insert it back into the device. Pour 500 g (1 lb 2 oz) of water into the mixer bowl. Place the beans into the simmering basket and insert into the mixer bowl. Cook for **10 min/steam mode/speed 2**, or until tender.

Meanwhile, heat the olive oil in a large frying pan over high heat. Season the steaks on both sides with sea salt and pepper. Cook the steaks for 2–3 minutes on each side for medium-rare, or until they are cooked to your liking. Remove from the pan and set aside to rest for 5 minutes.

Serve the steaks with the mash, beans and chimichurri.

GLUTEN-FREE | NUT-FREE | PALEO

AVOCADO PESTO PASTA SALAD WITH PRAWNS

Talk about a weeknight wonder! This is a fantastically easy and versatile recipe. The pesto for this can even be made in advance and kept in the fridge for up to 3 days, making it that much quicker to get on the table after a busy day.

SERVES 4

Preparation time 15 minutes
Cooking time 20 minutes

Pasta salad
375 g (13 oz) farfalle or rotelle pasta (or pasta of your choice)
350 g (12 oz) asparagus, trimmed and cut into 4 cm (1½ in) lengths
500 g (1 lb 2 oz) cooked peeled prawns, deveined and halved lengthways (you'll need to buy 1 kg/2 lb 4 oz of unpeeled prawns in order to get this much meat)

Avocado pesto
2 large handfuls basil leaves, plus extra small leaves to serve
1 small garlic clove
4 tablespoons pine nuts, toasted
2 tablespoons extra virgin olive oil
4 tablespoons lemon juice
1 large (250 g/9 oz) ripe avocado

Pour 1.25 kg (2 lb 12 oz) of water into the mixer bowl and season with salt. Bring the water to the boil for **8 min/100°C/speed 1** (without the measuring cup inserted into the lid).

Carefully, add the pasta to the mixer bowl. Attach the steaming basket instead of the measuring cup to the mixer bowl lid. Add the asparagus to the steaming basket and cook for **8 min/steam mode/reverse stir/speed 1** (or follow the timing given on the pasta packet). Cook until the pasta is al dente and the asparagus is tender, then drain both in a colander under running water. Transfer to a large bowl.

Next, make the pesto. Blend the basil leaves, garlic and half of the pine nuts with the oil, lemon juice and 1 tablespoon of water for **10 sec/speed 8**. Season well, then add the avocado and blend for **5 sec/speed 5**. Transfer to the bowl with the pasta and mix well to combine.

Serve the pasta with the prawns, remaining pine nuts and basil leaves.

DAIRY-FREE

TIP
You can swap steamed chicken breast for the prawns, or keep it simple and go vegetarian or vegan. I always buy unpeeled prawns as I think they are fresher and taste better.

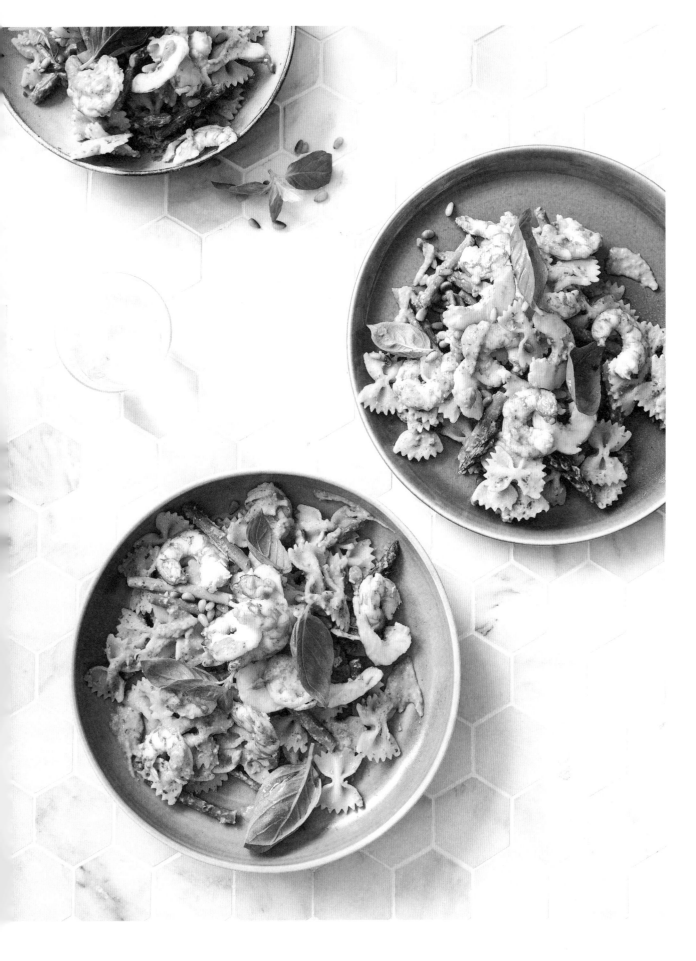

STEAMED SNAPPER WITH SICILIAN CAPONATA

Caponata sauce is great for busy families because it can be batch cooked, then frozen in airtight containers for up to 6 months. It goes really well with beef and chicken as well as fish and seafood. Feel free to vary the fish in this recipe, but keep an eye on cooking times as that will vary depending on which type of fish you use and the thickness of the fillets.

SERVES 4

Preparation time 10 minutes
Cooking time 20 minutes

1 red onion, peeled and quartered
1 eggplant (aubergine), cut into 3 cm (1¼ in) pieces
1 red capsicum (pepper), stem and seeds removed, cut into 3 cm (1¼ in) pieces
400 g (14 oz) Naked pasta sauce (page 14) or tinned chopped tomatoes
2 tablespoons extra virgin olive oil
1 handful basil leaves, torn
4 x 150 g (5½ oz) skinless baby snapper fillets
2 tablespoons baby capers, rinsed and drained
60 g (2¼ oz/⅓ cup) pitted Sicilian olives
2 tablespoons white wine vinegar
toasted pine nuts, to serve

Chop the onion for **5 sec/speed 5**. Scrape down the side of the bowl. Add the eggplant, capsicum, pasta sauce, 1 tablespoon of the oil and half of the basil. Season with salt and pepper. Cook for **8 min/120°C/ reverse stir/soft stir**.

Meanwhile, place the fish on the steaming tray then drizzle the remaining oil all over the fillets and season with salt and pepper.

Add the capers, olives and vinegar to the mixer bowl. Attach the empty steaming basket (with the tray of fish on top) to the mixer bowl lid. Cook for **8 min/steam mode/reverse stir/soft stir**, or until the fish is cooked.

Spoon the caponata sauce over the fish, then scatter over some pine nuts and the remaining basil leaves before serving.

MAKE AHEAD: FREEZE
DAIRY-FREE | GLUTEN-FREE | PALEO | LOW-CARB

CHAI-SPICED HONEY CHICKEN

Using chai tea to flavour the cooking liquid is an easy and subtle way to add some spice. This dish manages to be a great winter warmer without the heaviness of many traditional wintry dishes.

SERVES 4

Preparation time 10 minutes + standing time
Cooking time 20 minutes

200 g (7 oz/1 cup) quinoa (see Note)
2 garlic cloves
2 cm (¾ in) piece of ginger, peeled
750 ml (26 fl oz/3 cups) Chicken stock (page 31)
1 tablespoon raw honey
3 chai tea bags
1 teaspoon sea salt
2 x 300 g (10½ oz) skinless chicken breasts
400 g (14 oz) baby carrots, scrubbed or peeled, trimmed, leaving 2 cm (¾ in) tops attached
500 g (1 lb 2 oz) choy sum, trimmed, cut into 5 cm (2 in) lengths

Soak the quinoa in cold water for at least 30 minutes. Rinse well and drain.

Meanwhile, chop the garlic and ginger for **5 sec/speed 5**. Scrape down the side of the bowl. Add the stock, 200 g (7 oz) of water, honey, tea bags, quinoa and salt. Place the chicken and the carrots in the simmering basket and insert into the mixer bowl.

Place the choy sum stems in the steaming basket and the leaves on the steaming tray. Attach the steaming basket and tray, instead of the measuring cup, to the mixer bowl lid. Cook for **18 min/steam mode/ reverse stir/soft stir** until the chicken is cooked through and the quinoa and vegetables are tender.

Rest the chicken for 5 minutes before slicing, then serve with the quinoa, broth and vegetables.

DAIRY-FREE | GLUTEN-FREE | NUT-FREE | PALEO

NOTE

I soak quinoa in cold water for at least 30 minutes to wash away the bitter and soapy saponin on the exterior. If you leave your quinoa soaking for even longer, you may notice that some of the grains sprout, making it even better for you. If you want to sprout it, make sure to drain the soaking water after 12 hours and replace it with fresh water.

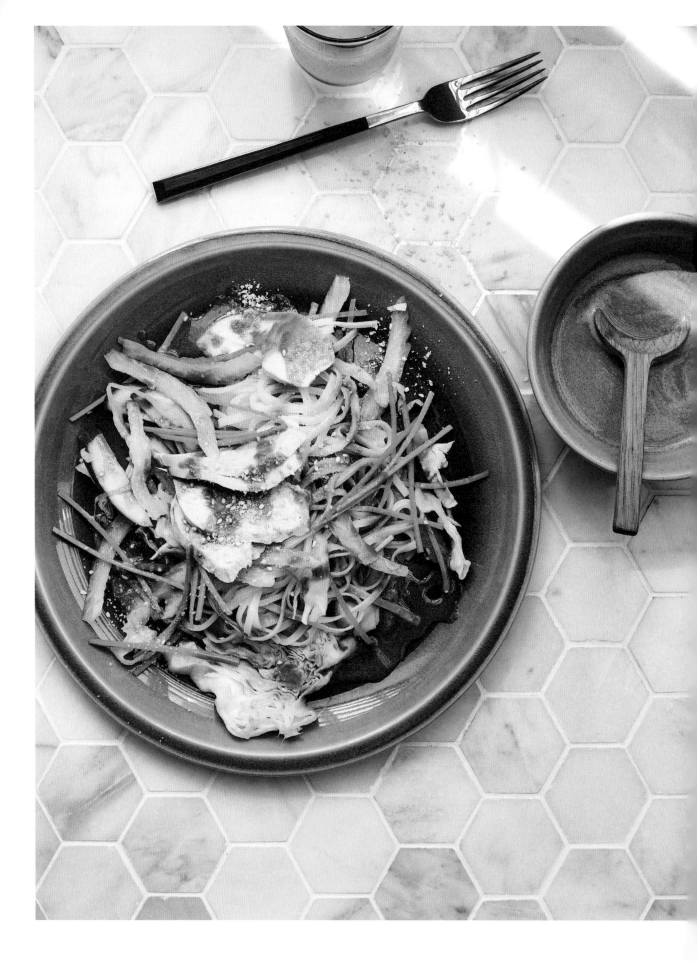

BANG BANG CHICKEN

If you are making tahini especially for this recipe, it's best to make it with *only* sesame oil, otherwise, you can find sesame paste in an Asian supermarket or use a store-bought tahini. If you prefer your bang bang sauce to have a milder chilli hit, halve the amount of chilli oil or completely replace it with sesame oil. Get ahead by making the sauce and storing it in the fridge for up to 5 days. Give it a good shake or stir before serving and you're good to go!

SERVES 4

Preparation time 15 minutes
Cooking time 20 minutes

125 ml (4 fl oz/½ cup) Tahini (page 39)
2 tablespoons Chinese black vinegar, rice or malt vinegar
3 tablespoons light soy sauce
1 tablespoon chilli oil or sesame oil
3 tablespoons maple syrup, rice syrup or sugar
2 x 250 g (9 oz) skinless chicken breasts
100 g (3½ oz) thin stick noodles

2 Lebanese (short) cucumbers, halved lengthways, thinly sliced on an angle
1 carrot, peeled and shredded or coarsely grated
½ iceberg lettuce, very thinly sliced
2 celery stalks, thinly sliced on an angle
Gomasio (page 39), to serve (optional)

Blend the tahini, vinegar, soy sauce, chilli oil and maple syrup for **10 sec/speed 8**. Transfer to a small bowl, then set aside.

Pour 500 g (1 lb 2 oz) of water into the mixer bowl. Place the chicken in the simmering basket and insert into the mixer bowl. Cook for **18 min/steam mode/speed 2**, or until cooked through. Carefully remove and set aside to rest for 5 minutes before thinly slicing.

Meanwhile, prepare the noodles according to the packet instructions, then drain well and cool. Combine the noodles with the salad ingredients in a large bowl and lightly toss everything together.

Serve the chicken and salad with the bang bang sauce drizzled on top and a sprinkling of gomasio, if using.

MAKE AHEAD: FRIDGE
DAIRY-FREE | PALEO

TIP

This can easily become a vegan dish if you serve the salad with steamed tofu instead of chicken.

CALIFORNIAN FISH TACOS

I've lost the battered fish and sour cream in my version of this Cali-Mex favourite. I love putting all the elements in the centre of the table and letting everyone make their own. My family loves adding extra jalapeños to their tacos, but add them to taste if you prefer less heat.

SERVES 4
Preparation time 15 minutes
Cooking time 10 minutes

1 handful coriander (cilantro), leaves picked, stems roughly chopped
10–20 g (¼–¾ oz) pickled jalapeño chillies, plus extra sliced chillies to serve
finely grated zest and juice of 1 lime
1 ripe avocado, stone removed, peeled
130 g (4¾ fl oz/½ cup) Labne (page 27) or thick Greek-style yoghurt
1 tablespoon neutral oil, such as grapeseed, rice bran or vegetable
2 teaspoons smoked paprika
4 x 150 g (5½ oz) boneless, skinless firm white fish fillets, such as barramundi
12 soft corn tortillas
1 tomato, quartered, seeds removed, cut into 1 cm (½ in) pieces
1 Lebanese (short) cucumber, halved lengthways, seeds removed, cut into 1 cm (½ in) pieces
170 g (6 oz) roasted red capsicum (pepper) strips

Chop the coriander stems and jalapeños for **5 sec/speed 5**. Scrape down the side of the bowl. Add the lime zest, avocado and labne, then season with salt and pepper. Blend for **10 sec/speed 5**. Transfer to a bowl and set aside.

Combine the oil and paprika in a bowl and season. Add the fish fillets and mix until well coated.

Pour 500 g (1 lb 2 oz) of water into the mixer bowl. Place the fish in the steaming basket. Cut out a baking paper round the same size as a tortilla. Place this in the centre of the steaming tray and place the tortillas on top. Attach the steaming basket and tray to the mixer bowl lid. Cook for **10 min/steam mode/speed 2**, or until the fish is cooked.

Meanwhile, combine the tomato, cucumber, capsicum, lime juice and coriander leaves in a bowl. Season and mix to combine. Serve the tortillas with chunks of the fish, guacamole, salsa and jalapeño slices.

GLUTEN-FREE | NUT-FREE

TIP

Using homemade labne instead of sour cream is one of the best tricks in the book if you're trying to make a few healthy swaps.

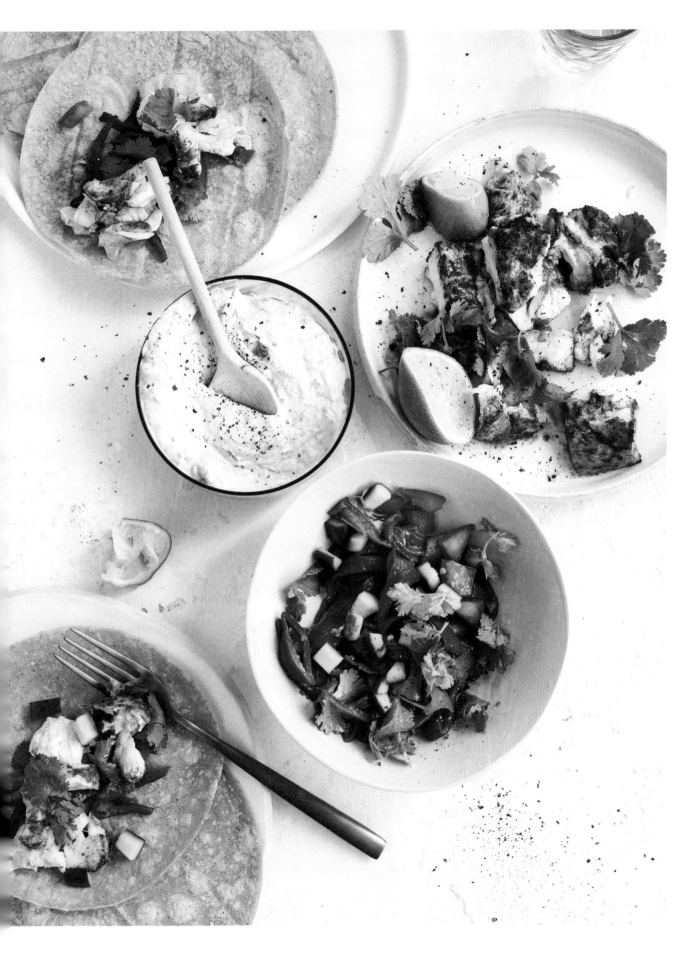

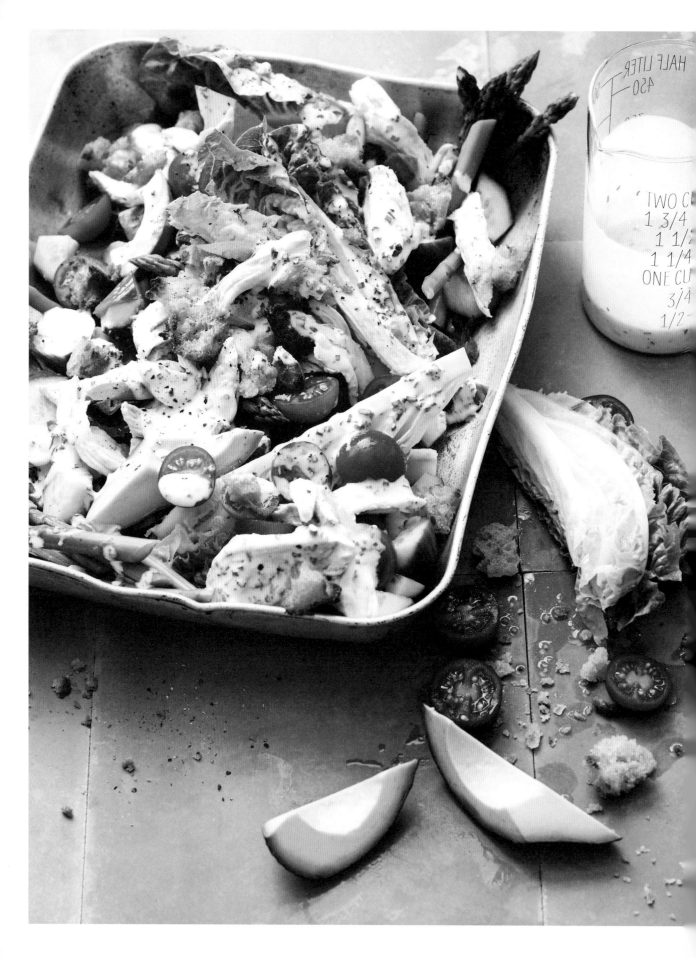

BEST CHICKEN SALAD

I know the title of this recipe is a big call, but I'm happy to stand by this claim.

SERVES 4
Preparation time 20 minutes
Cooking time 25 minutes

2 x 250 g (9 oz) chicken breasts
350 g (12 oz) asparagus trimmed and halved
300 g (10½ oz) No-work 'sourdough' (page 23), crust removed,
    torn into small pieces
extra virgin olive oil, to drizzle
2 tablespoons lemon juice
250 ml (9 fl oz/1 cup) Ranch dressing (page 47)
3 tablespoons finely chopped chives
2 teaspoons finely chopped tarragon, mint or parsley (optional)
2 baby cos (romaine) lettuces, trimmed and cut into thin wedges
2 Lebanese (short) cucumbers, roughly chopped
1 ripe avocado, stone removed, peeled and cut into wedges
250 g (9 oz) cherry tomatoes, halved

Preheat the oven to 200°C (400°F) and line a baking tray with baking paper. Pour 500 g (1 lb 2 oz) of water into the mixer bowl. Place the chicken in the simmering basket, insert into the mixer bowl and season with salt and pepper. Put the thicker ends of asparagus in the steaming basket and the spears in the steaming tray. Attach the steaming basket and tray to the mixer bowl lid. Cook for **10 min/steam mode/speed 2** until the asparagus is bright green and tender.

Remove the steaming basket and insert the measuring cup into the mixer bowl lid. Cook the chicken for a further **10 min/steam mode/ speed 2**, or until cooked through.

Meanwhile, put the bread chunks on the lined tray, drizzle with oil and toss to coat. Spread out in a single layer. Toast in the oven for 15 minutes, or until golden and crisp.

Transfer the chicken to a bowl and pour over the lemon juice. Set aside for 5 minutes to rest before shredding with two forks or slicing. Mix the ranch dressing, chives, tarragon, if using, and lemony resting juices together in a jug or bowl. Combine the salad ingredients and chicken in a large serving bowl then drizzle over the dressing just before serving.

NUT-FREE

TIP

Feel free to play around with the ingredients, this is a very forgiving salad. I love adding thinly sliced radishes to mine, and often swap in mint or parsley instead of tarragon. Use whatever you like and whatever is in your fridge.

FISH AND LEEK PIE WITH ROOT VEG MASH TOPPING

Pies are such a good way of sneaking as many veggies as possible into one mouthful. I tend to use a combination of parsnip and potato mash for the topping, to increase the goodness.

SERVES 4

Preparation time 15 minutes
Cooking time 30 minutes

30 g (1 oz) parmesan cheese, roughly chopped
2 leeks, white part only, washed and roughly chopped
30 g (1 oz) Butter (page 22)
2 tablespoons gluten-free or plain (all-purpose) flour
2 teaspoons Honey mustard (page 44) or dijon mustard
125 ml (4 fl oz/½ cup) Buttermilk (page 22) or milk

125 ml (4 fl oz/½ cup) Seafood, stock (page 33)
2 corn cobs, kernels removed
800 g (1 lb 12 oz) Root veg mash (page 42)
600 g (1 lb 5 oz) mix of boneless, skinless fish fillets, such as smoked cod, salmon and ling, diced into 3 cm (1¼ in) cubes
100 g (3½ oz) frozen peas
15 g (½ oz/½ cup) roughly chopped parsley

Preheat the oven to 220°C (425°F). Grate the parmesan for **15 sec/speed 10**. Transfer to a bowl and set aside.

Chop the leeks for **5 sec/speed 5**. Scrape down the side of the bowl. Add the butter and cook for **5 min/120°C/speed 1**.

Meanwhile, whisk the flour, mustard and buttermilk in a bowl. Add the flour mixture, stock and corn to the mixer bowl. Cook for **5 min/95°C/speed 2**. Combine half the parmesan with the mash in a bowl.

Transfer the mixture to a 2–2.5 litre (70–87 fl oz/8–10 cup) capacity pie or baking dish. Add the fish, peas and parsley, season with salt and pepper and gently mix to combine. Spoon and spread the mash over to cover, then scatter over the remaining parmesan.

Bake in the oven for 10 minutes, then switch the oven grill on and set it to high. Grill for 5 minutes, or until golden. Allow the pie to stand for 5 minutes before serving.

MAKE AHEAD: FREEZE
GLUTEN-FREE | NUT-FREE

TIP

You can make this pie ahead of time then wrap it up and pop it in the freezer for up to 3 months. If freezing, make sure all of the fish is fresh and wasn't frozen beforehand, and that the mash has completely cooled before you spoon it over the fish and peas.

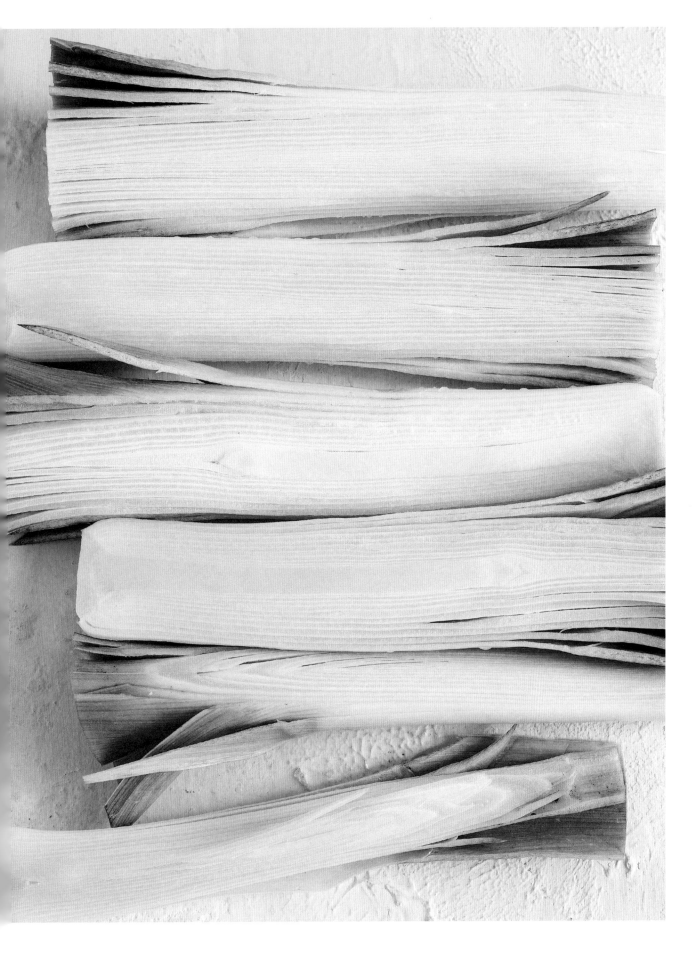

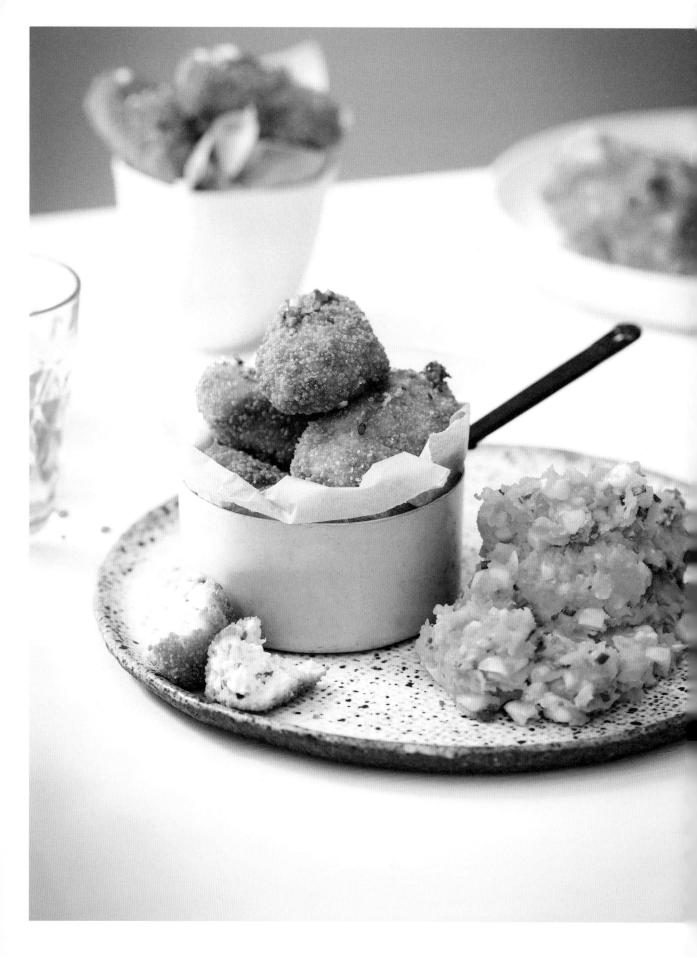

CHEESY CHICKEN NUGGETS WITH CORNY PUMPKIN MASH

These nuggets are deceptively good for the kids, and very popular at my house. To be extra-efficient, double the nugget recipe and freeze an uncooked batch in an airtight container (making sure the nuggets aren't touching) for up to 3 months.

SERVES 4

Preparation time 25 minutes
Cooking time 15 minutes

800 g (1 lb 12 oz) pumpkin mash
   (follow method on page 42)
2 garlic cloves, crushed
500 g (1 lb 2 oz) chicken tenderloins,
   roughly chopped
100 g (3½ oz) feta cheese
2 tablespoons finely chopped chives
1 egg white

1 teaspoon fine sea salt
2 corn cobs, kernels removed
50 g (1¾ oz/⅓ cup) plain
   (all-purpose) flour
255 g (9¼ oz/1⅓ cups) couscous
2 eggs, lightly beaten
olive oil, for frying

Preheat the oven to 120°C (235°F). Make the pumpkin mash then set aside and clean the mixer bowl out. Add the garlic, chicken, feta, chives, egg white and ½ teaspoon of the salt to the mixer bowl. Blend for **5 sec/ speed 5**. Shape heaped tablespoons of this mixture into nuggets.

Add 500 g (1 lb 2 oz) of water to the mixer bowl. Place the corn in the steaming basket and attach to the lid. Cook for **14 min/steam mode/ speed 3**. Place the flour, couscous and lightly beaten eggs into three separate shallow dishes. Coat the chicken pieces in the flour, shaking off any excess, then dip into the egg to coat, then into the couscous to coat.

Pour in enough oil to coat the base of a large frying pan and place over medium heat. In batches, cook the nuggets for 3–4 minutes, turning every 30 seconds, until golden and cooked through. Keep the first batch warm in the oven, while you cook the remaining nuggets.

To finish, blend the pumpkin mash and corn for **5 sec/speed 4**. Serve the nuggets with the mash and relish, if you like.

MAKE AHEAD: FREEZE

NUT-FREE | PALEO | LOW-CARB

TIP

To make this recipe gluten-free, you can substitute quinoa flakes or polenta (or a combination of the two) for the couscous, then use gluten-free plain flour to dust.

SALMON AND CUCUMBER TABBOULEH

If you're after a light, fresh and super-fast meal, this recipe ticks all of the boxes: time, ease of preparation and taste. It's a winner any night of the week.

SERVES 4

Preparation time 15 minutes + standing time
Cooking time 15 minutes

75 g (2¾ oz) fine burghul (bulgur) wheat
4 Lebanese (short) cucumbers, halved lengthways, seeds discarded and roughly chopped
1 small garlic clove (optional)
2 spring onions (scallions), cut into 2 cm (¾ in) lengths
4 large handfuls parsley leaves
2 large handfuls mint leaves
juice of 1–2 lemons (add to taste)
4 tablespoons extra virgin olive oil, plus extra to serve
4 x 150 g (5½ oz) boneless, skinless salmon fillets
sumac, for serving
50 g (1¾ oz) walnuts, toasted, roughly chopped, for serving
125 g (4 oz/½ cup) pomegranate seeds, for serving (optional)

Add the burghul to a large bowl and pour in 200 ml (7 fl oz) of boiling water to cover. Set aside for 20 minutes, or until tender and fluffy.

Meanwhile, chop the cucumber for **1–2 sec/speed 4**. Transfer to a large bowl. Chop the garlic, spring onions, parsley and mint for **3 sec/speed 6**.

Transfer the herb mixture to the bowl with the cucumbers. Stir in the lemon juice (add to taste), 3 tablespoons of the oil and burghul, season well with salt and pepper and mix until very well combined. Set aside.

Add 500 g (1 lb 2 oz) of water to the mixer bowl. Place the salmon into the steaming tray, drizzle with the remaining oil, season then sprinkle sumac over the surface. Attach the empty steaming basket and tray to the mixer bowl lid. Cook for **12 min/steam mode/speed 2** until the salmon is just cooked. Allow to cool, then separate into large chunks.

Top the tabbouleh with flaked salmon, walnuts, pomegranate seeds, if using, and a drizzle of extra virgin olive oil, then serve immediately.

DAIRY-FREE

TIP

You can easily make this recipe using quinoa instead of burghul to make it gluten-free. Add soaked quinoa to the simmering basket over 1 kg (2 lb 4 oz) of water and cook for **18 min/steam mode/ speed 3.**

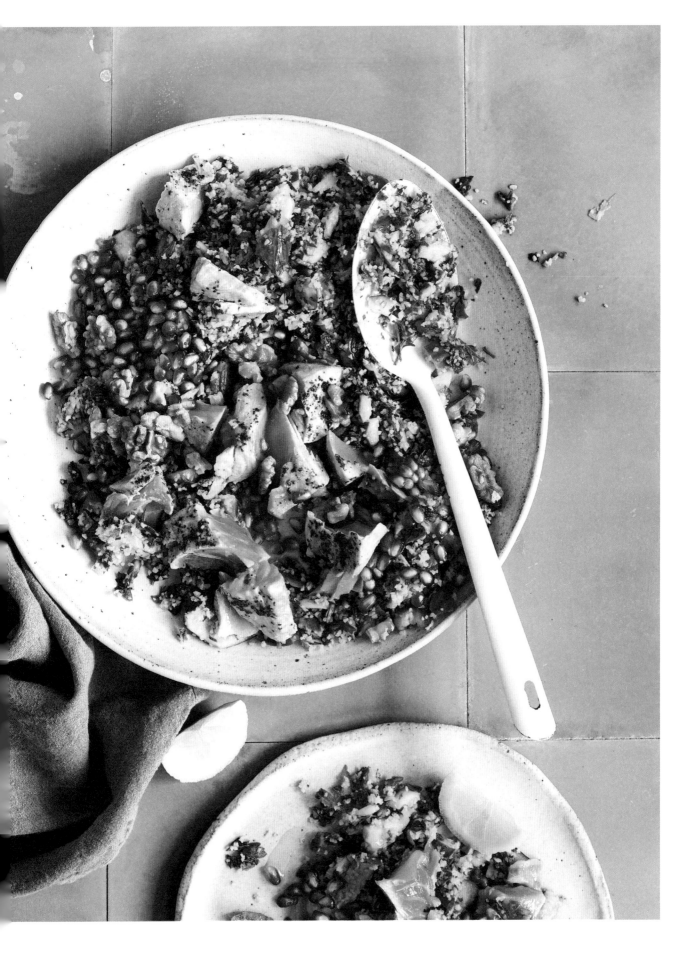

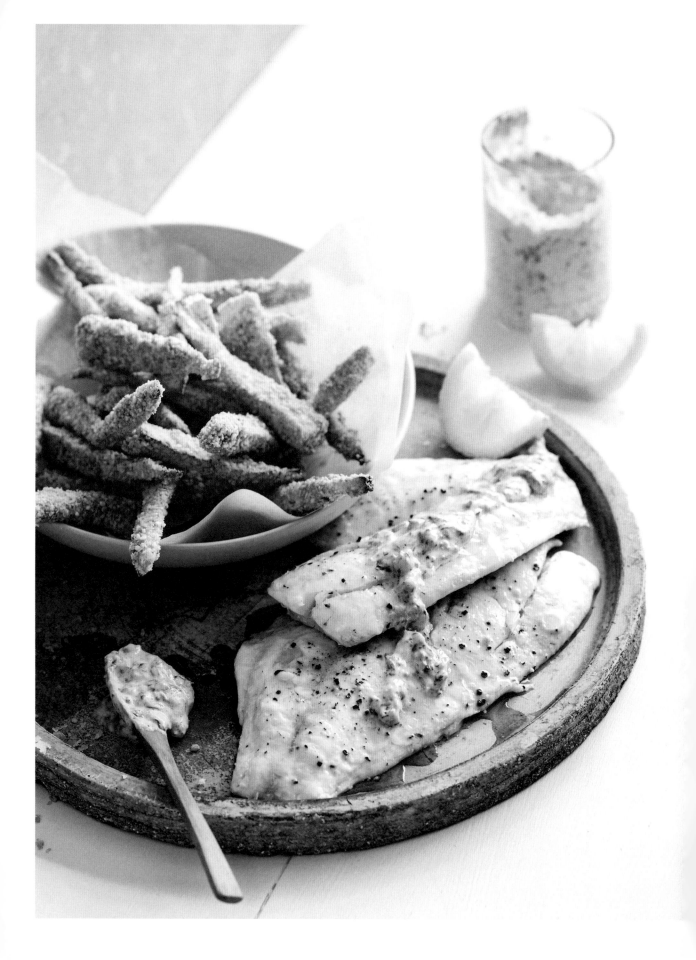

FISH AND CHIPS WITH YOGHURT TARTARE SAUCE

By swapping parsnips or sweet potatoes for potato chips and yoghurt for the tartare, this fish and chips meal is much lighter on the system but still tasty enough to keep everyone happy.

SERVES 4
Preparation time 15 minutes
Cooking time 20 minutes

Fish and chips
2 egg whites
180 g (6¼ oz/1½ cups) Gomasio (page 39)
1 kg (2 lb 4 oz) large parsnips, peeled and cored, cut into chip-sized pieces
olive oil or rice bran oil spray

Yoghurt tartare sauce
1–2 spring onions (scallions), roughly chopped
1 tablespoon capers, rinsed and drained
1 handful flat-leaf (Italian) parsley leaves
200 g (7 oz/¾ cup) Homemade yoghurt (made with cow's milk, page 26)
2 teaspoons lemon juice, plus wedges on the side
4 x 150 g (5½ oz) boneless, skinless fish fillets, such as baby snapper

Preheat the oven to 220°C (425°F) and line two baking trays with baking paper. Beat the egg whites for **1 min/speed 4**. Put the gomasio in a wide bowl and the egg whites in another wide bowl. Coat the chips in egg white, then in the gomasio and place in a single layer on the lined trays. Season with salt if the gomasio isn't seasoned and spray with oil.

Roast in the oven for 15–20 minutes until lightly golden and cooked, swapping the trays halfway through. Meanwhile, make your tartare sauce. Chop the spring onion, capers and parsley for **5 sec/speed 8**. Scrape down the side of the bowl. Add the yoghurt and lemon juice. Blend for **10 sec/speed 5**. Transfer to a bowl.

Add 500 g (1 lb 2 oz) of water to the mixer bowl. Place the fish onto the steaming tray and season with salt and pepper. Attach the empty steaming basket and tray to the mixer bowl lid. Cook for **10 min/ steam mode/speed 3**, or until just cooked through. Serve the fish with the chips and tartare sauce.

MAKE AHEAD: FRIDGE
GLUTEN-FREE

TIP

I'm partial to a little mustard in my tartare sauce. I find a teaspoon of Honey mustard (page 44) or dijon mustard added at the same time as the yoghurt and lemon juice adds an exciting background flavour.

THAI BEEF SALAD

Everyone in my family loves a Thai beef salad. Using sweet chilli sauce as part of the dressing is a good way to introduce Thai flavours if they're new to your family. The homemade version on page 46 isn't nearly as sweet as commercially made sauces, and it adds wonderful flavour to this salad. I prefer using sunflower seeds over the traditional peanut for this salad — they're a good source of many vitamins, especially vitamin E.

SERVES 4

Preparation time 20 minutes + standing time
Cooking time 10 minutes

200 g (7 oz) snow peas (mangetout), trimmed
500 g (1 lb 2 oz) rump steak
2 tablespoons sesame oil
125 ml (4 fl oz/½ cup) My not-too-sweet chilli sauce (page 46)
1 tablespoon gluten-free tamari (gluten-free soy sauce)
250 g (9 oz) cherry tomatoes, halved
2 Lebanese (short) cucumbers, roughly chopped
1 red capsicum (pepper), stem and seeds removed, cut into thin strips
1 carrot, peeled and shredded or coarsely grated
1 large handful of herbs: Thai basil, coriander (cilantro) and mint leaves
1 small red onion, halved and very thinly sliced
toasted sunflower seeds or slivered almonds, to serve

Add 500 g (1 lb 2 oz) of water to the mixer bowl. Place the snow peas into the simmering basket and insert into the mixer bowl. Cook for **6 min/ steam mode/speed 2** until bright green and tender. Rinse the snow peas under cold running water until cool to stop the cooking process.

Meanwhile, heat a frying pan over high heat. Drizzle the beef with 1 tablespoon of the sesame oil and season with salt and pepper on both sides. Cook the beef for 1–2 minutes on each side for rare, or until cooked to your liking. How long it takes will depend on the thickness of the steak. Set aside to rest for 5 minutes before slicing very thinly.

Meanwhile, combine the sweet chilli and soy sauces in a large bowl. Add all of the ingredients except the sunflower seeds and toss.

Serve the salad with sunflower seeds sprinkled on top.

DAIRY-FREE | GLUTEN-FREE | PALEO | LOW-CARB

CHEAT'S SAUSAGE CASSOULET

Sausages are a rare breed in my household, but everything in moderation is a much more sustainable approach when it comes to maintaining a healthy, balanced diet. There are lots of high-quality sausages available these days, but I still read through all of the ingredients on the label to make sure that the meat content is high enough. Generally speaking, 65–70% is a good start, but the higher, the better. I also check that there aren't too many other ingredients – especially ones I don't recognise!

SERVES 4

Preparation time 10 minutes
Cooking time 20 minutes

1 onion, peeled and halved
1 tablespoon olive oil
2 teaspoons gluten-free or plain (all-purpose) flour
2 carrots, peeled, quartered and cut into 1.5 cm (⅝ in) pieces
500 ml (17 fl oz/2 cups) Vegetable or Chicken stock (pages 32 and 31)
500 g (1 lb 2 oz) cooked cannellini beans or 2 x 400 g (14 oz) tins, rinsed and drained
2 tablespoons thyme leaves
500 g (1 lb 2 oz) gluten-free Italian sausages
400 g (14 oz) silverbeet (Swiss chard), thinly sliced, including the stems

Chop the onion for **5 sec/speed 5**. Scrape down the side of the bowl. Add the oil and sprinkle over the flour. Cook for **3 min/120°C/speed 1**.

Add the carrot, stock, beans and thyme and season with salt and pepper. Squeeze the sausages out of their skins into bite-sized pieces into the simmering basket. Place the silverbeet stems into the steaming basket and the leaves onto the steaming tray. Attach the steaming basket and tray, instead of the measuring cup, to the mixer bowl lid. Cook for **15 min/steam mode/reverse stir/soft stir**.

Carefully add the sausage pieces to the mixer bowl and mix for **1 min/ reverse stir/speed 1**.

Divide the silverbeet between your serving bowls and top with the cassoulet to serve.

GLUTEN-FREE | NUT-FREE

OREGANO LAMB WITH BEETROOT TZATZIKI

This is one of those clever dishes that looks a little fancy, but is actually easy to bring together. A real crowd pleaser.

SERVES 4

Preparation time 15 minutes
Cooking time 20 minutes

Beetroot tzatziki
1 small garlic clove
1 Lebanese (short) cucumber, roughly chopped
390 g (13¾ oz/1½ cups) Homemade yoghurt (page 26)
1½ teaspoons fine sea salt
500 g (1 lb 2 oz) beetroot, peeled and cut into 2.5 cm (1 in) pieces

Oregano lamb
2 tablespoons olive oil
1 tablespoon dried oregano
1 lemon, zest finely grated, cut into wedges
500 g (1 lb 2 oz) Frenched lamb cutlets
1 large handful mint leaves

Chop the garlic for **5 sec/speed 5**. Add the cucumber and chop for **5 sec/speed 4**. Transfer to a clean tea towel and squeeze out as much excess liquid as possible. Combine the yoghurt, 1 teaspoon of the salt and the cucumber mixture in a bowl. Line a sieve with paper towel and set inside a bowl or jug. Transfer the yoghurt mixture to the sieve and place in the fridge until needed.

Add 750 g (1 lb 10 oz) of water to the mixer bowl. Place the beetroot into the simmering basket and insert into the mixer bowl. Cook for **20 min/steam mode/speed 3**, or until almost tender.

Combine the oil, oregano and lemon zest in a bowl and season with salt and pepper. Add the lamb and mix until well coated. Heat a large frying pan over medium–high heat. In batches, cook the cutlets for 2 minutes each side for medium–rare or until cooked to your liking. Remove, set aside to rest for 2 minutes and keep warm.

Meanwhile, chop the beetroot for **5 sec/speed 4**. Discard any liquid that has strained from the yoghurt mixture into the bowl. Add the yoghurt mixture to the mixer bowl and mix for **10 sec/speed 3**.

Serve the lamb with the tzatziki, mint and lemon wedges.

MAKE AHEAD: FRIDGE

GLUTEN-FREE | NUT-FREE | PALEO | LOW-CARB

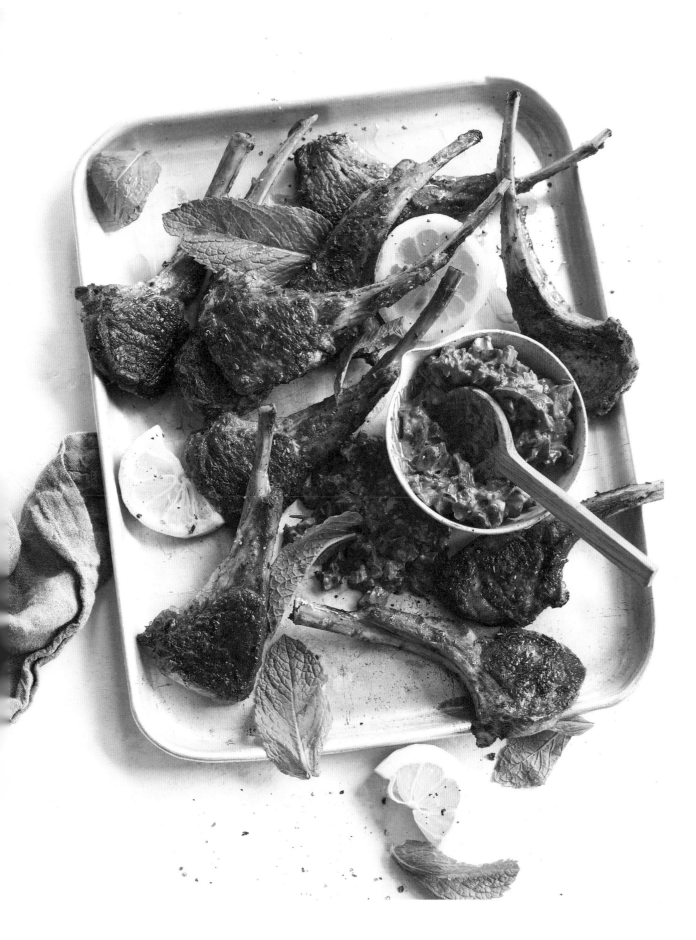

LAMB BOLOGNESE

I love using anchovies to add flavour to dishes, especially lamb dishes. They end up melting into the background, and don't make the meal fishy in any way. I always make a double batch because this freezes really well and keeps for up to 6 months. It's a lifesaver if you find yourself hosting a crowd. You can also use this recipe for the moussaka (page 152) in place of the mushroom and lentil mixture or in the lasagne (page 160).

SERVES 4
Preparation time 10 minutes
Cooking time 35 minutes

30 g (1 oz) parmesan cheese, roughly chopped
1 red onion, peeled and quartered
2 carrots, peeled and roughly chopped
2 celery stalks, roughly chopped
4 anchovy fillets
1 tablespoon extra virgin olive oil, plus extra to serve
500 g (1 lb 2 oz) minced (ground) lamb
400 g (14 oz) Naked pasta sauce (page 14) or
    tinned chopped tomatoes
¼ teaspoon dried chilli flakes
400 g (14 oz) pappardelle pasta
chopped parsley, to serve (optional)

Grate the parmesan for **15 sec/speed 10**. Transfer to a small bowl.

Chop the onion, carrot, celery and anchovies for **4 sec/speed 5**. Scrape down the side of the bowl. Add the oil and the lamb, and cook for **5 min/120°C/speed 1**.

Add the pasta sauce and chilli flakes and cook for **30 min/100°C/ reverse stir/soft stir**.

Meanwhile, bring a large saucepan of salted water to the boil. Cook the pasta according to the packet instructions until al dente. Drain and keep warm.

Serve the pasta with a generous spoonful of bolognese and sprinkle over some grated parmesan and parsley, if using. Finish with a drizzle of extra virgin olive oil.

MAKE AHEAD: FREEZE
NUT-FREE

GREEN MAC 'N' CHEESE

I don't like to waste any part of a vegetable if it can be eaten, and broccoli stems are no exception. I always peel the tough outer skin off the stem then dice it and cook it along with the florets. The same goes for cauliflower. This is another very versatile recipe; you can use any other nuts you like in place of the pine nuts, and other herbs such as basil, coriander or a combination, depending on what you have in your fridge.

SERVES 4

Preparation time 10 minutes
Cooking time 20 minutes

25 g (1 oz) parmesan cheese, roughly chopped (see Note on page 36)
2 large handfuls roughly chopped parsley, including the stems
1 small garlic clove
80 g (2¾ oz/½ cup) pine nuts, toasted (toasting is optional)
2 tablespoons extra virgin olive oil
2 tablespoons lemon juice
350 g (12 oz) broccoli, stem peeled and roughly chopped
400 g (14 oz) macaroni pasta
1 quantity cauliflower bechamel (page 36), warm

Grate the parmesan for **15 sec/speed 10**. Transfer to a bowl and set aside.

Add the parsley, garlic, most of the pine nuts, the oil and lemon juice to the mixer bowl, then season. Blend for **15 sec/speed 7**. Transfer to a bowl and set aside.

Chop the broccoli for **5 sec/speed 5**. Transfer to the steaming basket.

Pour 1.25 kg (2 lb 12 oz) of water into the mixer bowl and season. Bring to the boil for **10 min/100°C/speed 1** without the measuring cup inserted into the lid. Carefully, add the pasta to the mixer bowl. Attach the steaming basket to the mixer bowl lid. Cook for **6 min/steam mode/ reverse stir/speed 2**, or until the pasta is al dente and the broccoli is tender. Drain the pasta in a colander.

Add the broccoli, pesto, pasta and bechamel to the mixer bowl. Cook for **2 min/100°C/reverse stir/speed 2** until well combined.

Serve the pasta with the grated parmesan and remaining pine nuts.

VEGETARIAN

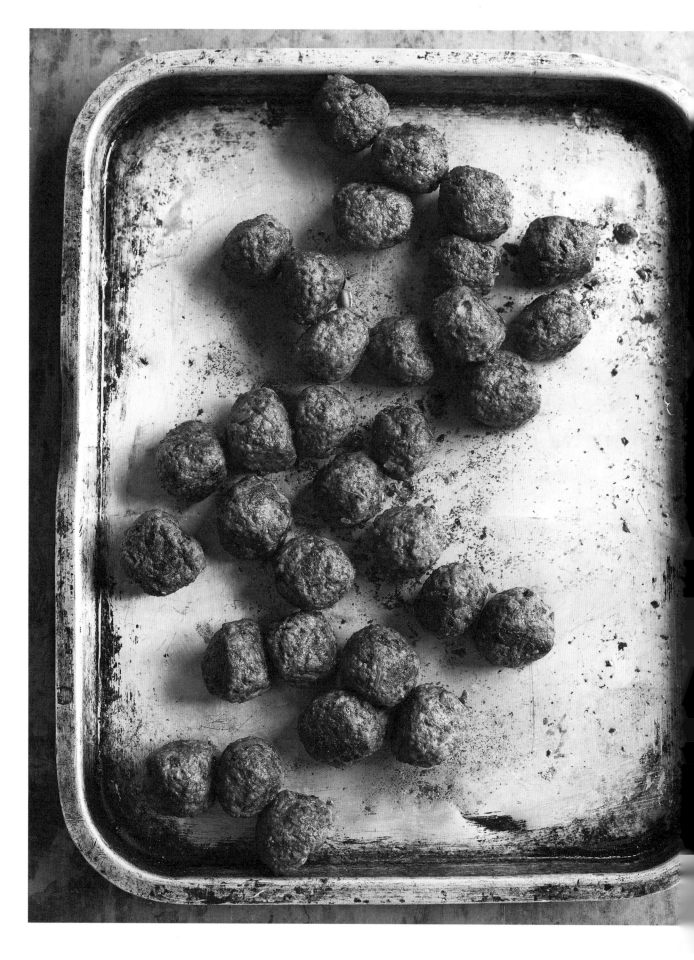

MEXICAN MEATBALL TACOS

There are lots of different Mexican spice blends available, so if yours is particularly spicy, start with a little and add more to taste.

SERVES 4

Preparation time 20 minutes
Cooking time 10 minutes

30 g (1 oz) coriander (cilantro)
1 ripe avocado, stone removed, peeled
2 tablespoons lime juice
1 zucchini (courgette), roughly chopped
500 g (1 lb 2 oz) minced (ground) beef
1–2 tablespoons Mexican spice blend (see recipe intro)
400 g (14 oz) Naked pasta sauce (page 14) or tinned chopped tomatoes
1 x 400 g (14 oz) tin kidney beans, rinsed and drained
12 corn tortillas
1 tablespoon olive oil

Chop the top half of the coriander for **3 sec/speed 5**. Add the avocado and lime juice and season with salt. Blend for **3 sec/speed 5**. Transfer to a bowl, then wash and dry the mixer bowl.

Chop the coriander stems and zucchini for **5 sec/speed 5**. Scrape down the side of the bowl and insert the whisk attachment. Add the minced beef, half the spice blend and season with sea salt. Mix for **2 min/speed 2** until well combined. Roll the mixture into 3 cm (1¼ in) balls.

Add the pasta sauce, remaining spice mix and kidney beans to the unwashed bowl. Cut out a piece of baking paper which is the size of one tortilla. Place the baking paper circle into the centre of the steaming tray and place the tortillas on top. Attach the empty steaming basket and tray, instead of the measuring cup, to the mixer bowl lid. Cook for **10 min/steam mode/reverse stir/speed 1**.

Meanwhile, heat the oil in a large frying pan over medium heat. Cook the meatballs for 6–8 minutes, turning regularly until golden and cooked through. Pour the sauce into the pan and mix to combine.

Pop two or three meatballs in each tortilla then top with guacamole and sauce.

MAKE AHEAD: FREEZE
DAIRY-FREE | GLUTEN-FREE | NUT-FREE

TIP

These tacos are a real family favourite, so it's worth making more than you need and freezing them, uncooked, for up to 3 months.

ITALIAN BRAISED BEAN AND 'POTATO' PASTA

The flavour of Jerusalem artichokes is so unique and delicious, that whenever they are in season, they are a must-have in my home. The great thing is, they can pass as potatoes, so they're yet another sneaky way of introducing a new vegetable to any fussy eaters. You can also use potatoes or standard marinated artichokes in this dish, if you prefer. If you want to use your mixer to cook the pasta, cook it before you cook the sauce. Angel hair pasta doesn't take very long which is why I like to cook it at the same time as the sauce.

SERVES 4

Preparation time 10 minutes
Cooking time 30 minutes

50 g (1¾ oz) parmesan cheese (see Note on page 36)
1 tablespoon extra virgin olive oil, plus extra to serve
300 g (10½ oz) Jerusalem artichokes or waxy potatoes,
    peeled and cut into 2.5 cm (1 in) pieces
400 g (14 oz) green beans, trimmed
800 g (1 lb 12 oz) Naked pasta sauce (page 14) or tinned chopped tomatoes
2 tablespoons baby capers, rinsed and drained
1 large handful basil leaves, plus extra to serve
375 g (13 oz) long pasta, such as angel hair

Grate the parmesan for **15 sec/speed 10**. Transfer to a bowl and set aside.

Add the oil, artichokes, beans, pasta sauce, capers and basil to the mixer bowl and season with salt and pepper. Cook for **30 min/100°C/ reverse stir/soft stir** until the artichokes are tender.

Meanwhile, bring a large saucepan of salted water to the boil. Cook the pasta according to the packet instructions. Drain then return the pasta to the pan.

Add the pasta sauce to the pasta and mix until well combined.

Serve with the grated parmesan, basil leaves and extra virgin olive oil.

NUT-FREE | VEGETARIAN

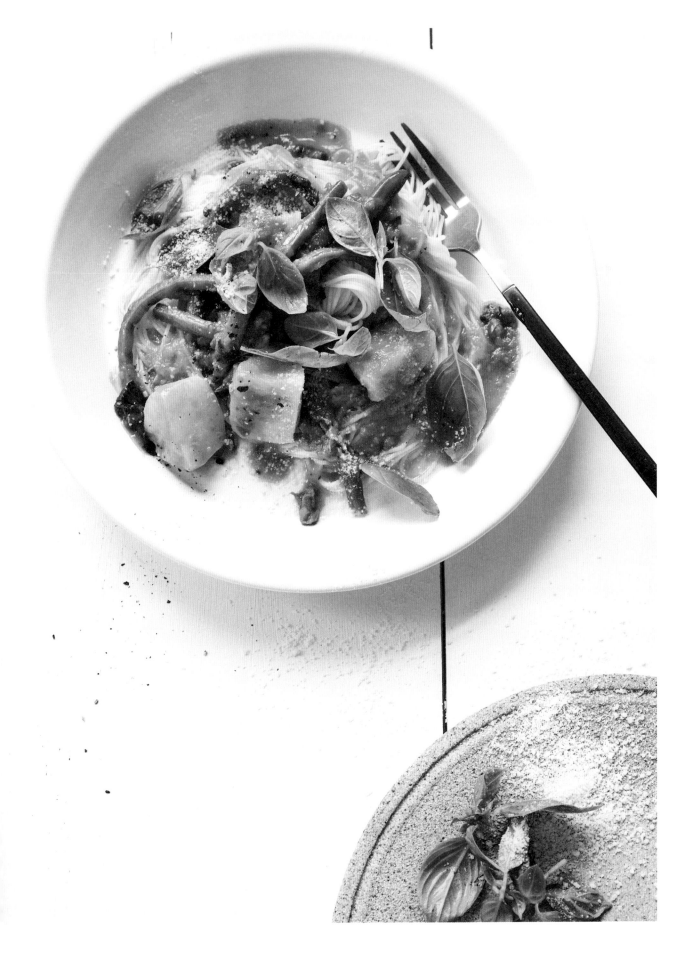

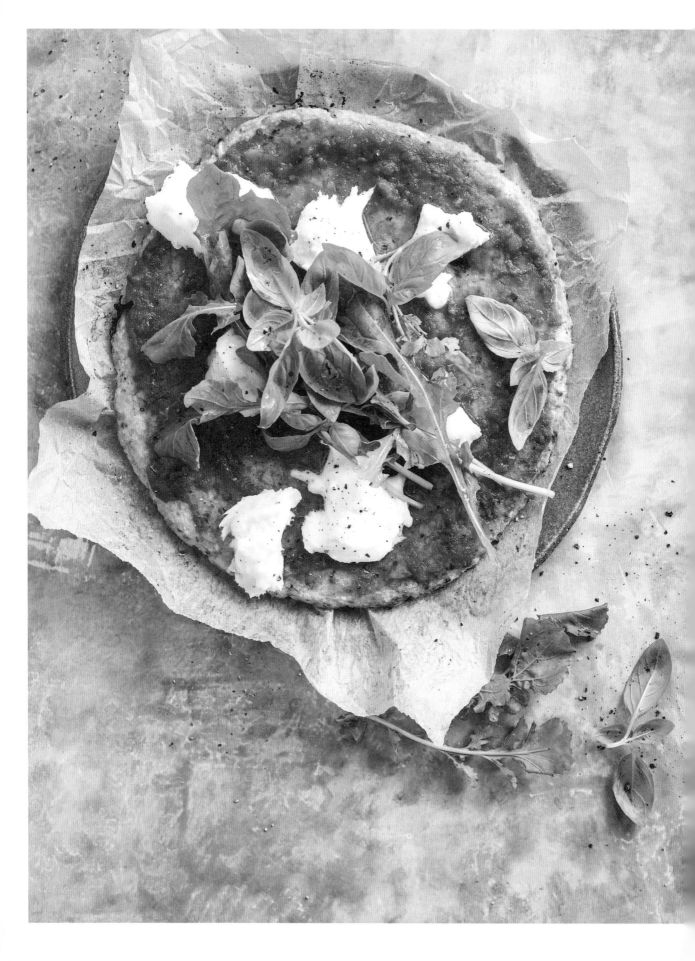

CAULIFLOWER PIZZA

What's not to like about cauliflower pizza? The base isn't fragile, it's an easy way to get more vegetables into the meal, and it tastes better than a lot of the gluten-free options I've tried – it's a win-win! It's surprising just how strong the base is, so feel free to get creative and load up the toppings.

MAKES 2
Preparation time 20 minutes + standing time
Cooking time 35 minutes

1 kg (2 lb 4 oz) cauliflower, cut into florets
50 g (1¾ oz) parmesan cheese (see Note on page 36)
1 teaspoon dried herbs such as oregano, Italian herbs or rosemary (optional)
2 eggs
a pinch of dried chilli flakes (optional)
1 quantity Pizza sauce (page 15)
1 buffalo mozzarella ball
1 large handful basil leaves
200 g (7 oz) rocket (arugula) leaves

Preheat the oven to 220°C (425°F) and line two baking trays with baking paper.

Chop the cauliflower in batches for **5 sec/speed 5**. Transfer to the simmering basket. Add 500 g (1 lb 2 oz) of water to the mixer bowl, then insert the simmering basket into the mixer bowl. Cook for **10 min/steam mode/speed 3** until the cauliflower is cooked. Transfer to a clean tea towel and allow to cool. Squeeze out as much excess water as possible.

Grate the parmesan for **15 sec/speed 5**. Scrape down the side of the bowl. Add the cauliflower, dried oregano, eggs, chilli flakes, if using, and season with sea salt and pepper. Mix for **30 sec/speed 3**.

Shape the cauliflower mixture into two rounds about 8 mm (⅜ in) thick on each lined tray. Bake in the oven for 20 minutes, swapping the shelves halfway through.

Spread the pizza sauce on the bases and cook them in the oven for a further 5 minutes. Remove from the oven, tear over the mozzarella. then top with the basil and rocket leaves. Finish with a drizzle of extra virgin olive oil and a pinch of salt and pepper, then serve.

MAKE AHEAD: FREEZE
GLUTEN-FREE | NUT-FREE | PALEO | VEGETARIAN

TIP
Though the base for these pizzas does take a little longer to make, they freeze really well so are a brilliant thing to stock up on. Pop them in the fridge to defrost the night before you want to serve them, then top and cook for a super-easy dinner.

VEGETABLE GREEN CURRY WITH NOODLES

I particularly love noodles with green curry, but brown or white rice would also do the trick. Balance the flavours to your taste, especially when it comes to adding the fish sauce.

SERVES 4

Preparation time 20 minutes
Cooking time 20 minutes

30 g (1 oz) palm sugar (jaggery), rice syrup or raw sugar
1 carrot, peeled and roughly chopped
1 tablespoon coconut oil
50 g (1¾ oz) green curry paste
2 x 400 ml (14 fl oz) tins coconut milk
120 g (4¼ oz) baby corn, halved lengthways
1 x 225 g (8 oz) tin bamboo shoot strips, drained

200 g (7 oz) fried tofu puffs, halved into triangles
250 g (9 oz) broccoli, cut into small florets
150 g (5½ oz) snow peas (mangetout), trimmed
2–3 tablespoons fish sauce
2 tablespoons lime juice, plus wedges to serve
200 g (7 oz) thin rice noodles
Thai basil leaves, to serve

Grate the palm sugar for **10 sec/speed 10**. Remove and set aside. Chop the carrot for **2 sec/speed 5**. Remove and set aside.

Add the coconut oil and curry paste to the mixer bowl. Cook for **3 min/120°C/speed 1**. Add the coconut milk, then fill one tin with water and pour into the mixer bowl. Add the carrot and baby corn. Cook for **5 min/95°C/reverse stir/soft stir**.

Meanwhile, add the broccoli to the simmering basket and the snow peas to the steaming basket. After the carrot has been cooking for 5 minutes, add the bamboo strips and tofu to the mixer bowl. Attach the steaming basket, instead of the measuring cup, to the mixer bowl lid. Cook for **10 min/steam mode/reverse stir/soft stir**.

Add the fish sauce, lime juice and sugar to the mixer bowl. Re-attach the steaming basket to the mixer bowl lid. Cook for **2 min/steam mode/ reverse stir/soft stir**. Cook the noodles according to packet instructions.

Serve the curry with the noodles, basil leaves and lime wedges.

DAIRY-FREE | GLUTEN-FREE | NUT-FREE

TUNA PUTTANESCA PASTA

This quick, easy and light pasta is my husband's go-to dish, and one that we all enjoy. The pasta cooking time given below is only a guide, you're always best to follow the timings on the packet instructions. Alternatively, you can boil the pasta in a saucepan to speed up the cooking process, while you cook the sauce in your mixer and it will be on the table in half the time.

SERVES 4

Preparation time 10 minutes
Cooking time 30 minutes

400 g (14 oz) short pasta, such as ditali
1 long red chilli, stem and seeds removed
3 garlic cloves
4 anchovy fillets
1 tablespoon extra virgin olive oil, plus extra to serve
425 g (15 oz) tuna chunks in oil, drained
400 g (14 oz) Naked pasta sauce (page 14) or tinned chopped tomatoes
2 tablespoons baby capers, rinsed and drained
15 g (½ oz/½ cup) finely chopped parsley
finely grated zest of 1 lemon

Add 1.25 kg (2 lb 12 oz) of water to the mixer bowl and season with salt. Bring the water to the boil for **10 min/100°C/speed 1** without the measuring cup inserted into the lid. Carefully, add the pasta to the mixer bowl. Cook for **10 min/100°C/reverse stir/speed 1** until the pasta is al dente. Drain the pasta in a colander and keep warm.

Chop the chilli, garlic and anchovies for **5 sec/speed 5**. Add the oil and cook for **2 min/120°C/reverse stir/speed 2**.

Add the tuna, pasta sauce and capers and season with salt and pepper. Cook for **5 min/120°C/reverse stir/soft stir** until hot.

Serve the pasta with the sauce, parsley, lemon zest and olive oil.

DAIRY-FREE

ORANGE RISOTTO

I find adding a vegetable purée to a risotto is a much better and easier way to add flavour and depth to your risotto, rather than simply relying on stock. Crumbled goat's cheese, feta, or grated haloumi are great alternatives to ricotta if you don't have any on hand.

SERVES 4
Preparation time 10 minutes
Cooking time 45 minutes

30 g (1 oz) parmesan cheese, roughly chopped (see Note on page 36)
2 carrots, peeled and roughly chopped
400 g (14 oz) peeled pumpkin, cut into 2.5 cm (1 in) pieces
1 litre (35 fl oz/4 cups) Vegetable or Chicken stock (pages 32 or 31)
1 onion, peeled and quartered
2 garlic cloves
1 tablespoon extra virgin olive oil, plus extra to serve
300 g (10½ oz) arborio rice
1 tablespoon thyme leaves
200 g (7 oz) fresh ricotta cheese

Grate the parmesan for **15 sec/speed 10**. Transfer to a small bowl. Chop the carrot for **3 sec/speed 5**. Transfer to a bowl and keep warm.

Add the pumpkin and stock to the mixer bowl. Cook for **12–15 min/ 100°C/speed 1**. Blend for **20 sec/speed 6** until smooth. Transfer to a jug or bowl.

Chop the onion and garlic for **5 sec/speed 5**. Scrape down the side of the bowl. Add the oil and cook for **3 min/120°C/speed 1**.

Insert the whisk attachment and add the rice, thyme and carrot. Cook for **1 min/120°C/reverse stir/speed 1**. Scrape down the side of the bowl. Add the pumpkin purée. Cook for **20–25 min/110°C/reverse stir/ speed 1** until the rice is al dente.

Add the grated parmesan and half the ricotta, then season well with salt and pepper. Cook for **1 min/110°C/speed 2**.

Serve the risotto with the remaining ricotta crumbled on top and a drizzle of extra virgin olive oil.

GLUTEN-FREE | NUT-FREE | VEGETARIAN

TIP

If I'm not worried about making this nut-free, I also like adding some roughly chopped nuts just before serving. Their texture and crunch provide a wonderful contrast to the creamy risotto.

GREEN RISOTTO

Like the orange risotto next door, the veg and herbs that get blended up here are a great way of boosting the average risotto's flavour profile, while also providing any vegetable-challenged family members with a dose of green. Once again, feel free to change the cheese or nuts to suit your taste.

SERVES 4

Preparation time 15 minutes
Cooking time 35 minutes

50 g (1¾ oz) parmesan, roughly chopped (see Note on page 36)
1 leek, white part only, washed and roughly chopped
2 garlic cloves
20 g (¾ oz) Butter (page 22)
250 g (9 oz) English spinach washed well, roughly chopped (including stems)
1 large handful basil or parsley leaves
250 g (9 oz) frozen peas
1 tablespoon extra virgin olive oil, plus extra to drizzle
300 g (10½ oz) arborio rice
750 ml (26 fl oz/3 cups) hot Vegetable or Chicken stock (pages 32 and 31)
50 g (1¾ oz) toasted pistachios or pine nuts

Grate the parmesan for **15 sec/speed 10**. Transfer to a small bowl. Chop the leek and garlic for **5 sec/speed 5**. Scrape down the side of the bowl. Add the butter and cook for **3 min/120°C/speed 1**.

Add the spinach and half the basil and chop for **4 sec/speed 5**. Scrape down the side of the bowl. Cook for **2 min/120°C/speed 1**. Add one-third of the peas and cook for **2 min/120°C/speed 1**. Season with salt and pepper and blend for **20 sec/speed 8**. Transfer to a bowl and set aside. Don't wash the bowl.

Insert the whisk attachment, then add the oil and rice. Cook for **1 min/120°C/reverse stir/speed 1**. Scrape down the side of the bowl. Add the hot stock and cook for **20–25 min/110°C/reverse stir/speed 1** until the rice is al dente. Meanwhile, combine the remaining peas, purée and parmesan in a bowl. After the risotto has been cooking for 20 minutes, add the green mixture and cook for **3 min/100°C/speed 1**.

Serve the risotto with the remaining basil leaves and pistachios scattered on top and a drizzle of extra virgin olive oil.

GLUTEN-FREE | VEGETARIAN

SESAME-CRUSTED TOFU WITH SWEET CHILLI NOODLES

Gomasio is such a great ingredient to use as a crust, especially with silky-soft silken tofu. A crunchy top and bottom is all you need, so don't worry too much about coating the sides.

SERVES 4

Preparation time 15 minutes + standing time
Cooking time 25 minutes

600 g (1 lb 5 oz) silken tofu, drained and cut into four rectangular 'steaks'
350 g (12 oz) dried soba noodles (use the timing on the packet instructions)
4 tablespoons black or white Gomasio (page 39) or sesame seeds
400 g (14 oz) baby carrots, peeled and sliced on an angle
175 g (6 oz) broccolini, cut into thirds
300 g (10½ oz) sugar snap peas, strings removed
2 tablespoons sesame oil
4 tablespoons My not-too-sweet chilli sauce (page 46)
1 tablespoon soy sauce

Add 1.25 kg (2 lb 12 oz) of water to the mixer bowl. Bring the water to the boil for **8–10 min/100°C/speed 1** without the measuring cup inserted into the lid. Carefully, add the soba noodles and cook for **4 min/100°C/reverse stir/speed 2**, or until the noodles are al dente. Drain well and rinse under cold running water until cool, then set aside.

Put the gomasio in a shallow dish or plate. Carefully coat the top and bottom of each tofu steak in the gomasio. Set aside.

Add 500 g (1 lb 2 oz) of water to the mixer bowl. Place the carrot into the simmering basket and insert into the mixer bowl. Add the broccolini to the steaming basket and the sugar snap peas to the steaming tray. Attach the steaming basket and tray, instead of the measuring cup, to the mixer bowl lid. Cook for **10 min/steam mode/reverse stir/speed 1**.

Meanwhile, heat 1 tablespoon of the oil in a large, non-stick frying pan over medium heat. Add the tofu and cook for 2 minutes each side, or until golden and toasted. Remove, set aside and keep warm. Reduce the heat to low. Add the remaining oil, sweet chilli and soy sauces and stir to combine. Heat for 1 minute, then add the noodles and vegetables and toss to combine. Cook for 1–2 minutes until heated through then serve right away with the warm crispy tofu.

DAIRY-FREE | VEGAN

TIP
Drain the tofu well before using and pat it dry with paper towel. I often leave my tofu wrapped in paper towel sitting on a plate for at least 5 minutes, to absorb as much water as possible.

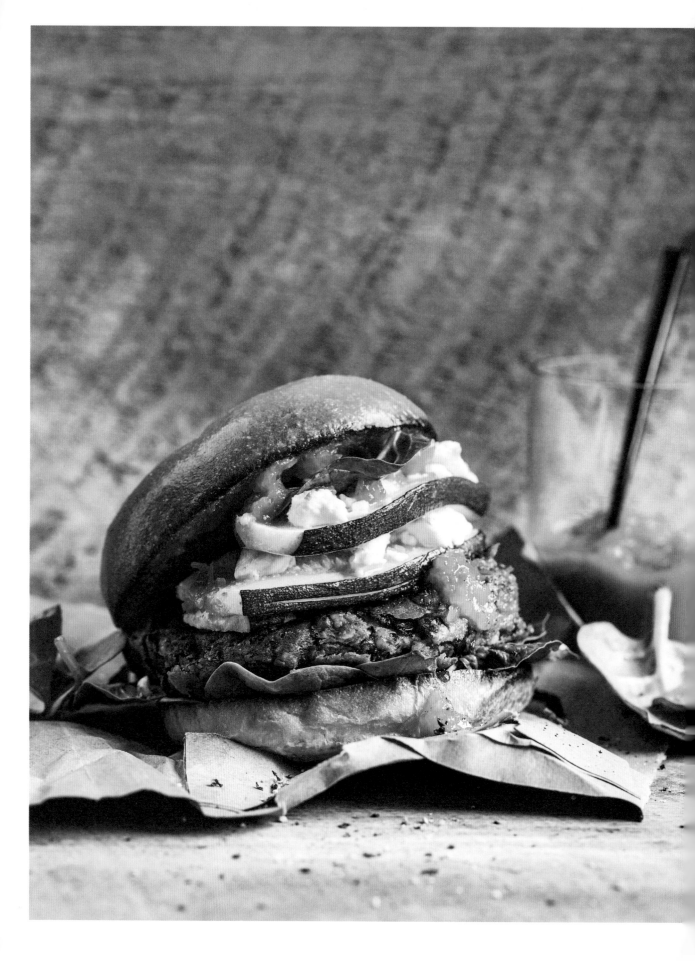

ULTIMATE VEGGIE BURGERS

Veggie burgers get a bad rap because there are some pretty bad ones around. But I guarantee you won't feel like you're missing out with these 'meaty' patties. They're so good, you'll be calling up all your veggie friends to rave about them.

SERVES 4

Preparation time 15 minutes
Cooking time 10 minutes

2 garlic cloves
100 g (3½ oz) walnuts
2 x 400 g (14 oz) tins kidney beans, rinsed and drained
50 g (1¾ oz) buckwheat or chickpea flour (besan)
1 egg
30 g (1 oz/½ cup) roughly chopped basil or flat-leaf (Italian) parsley
150 g (5½ oz) feta cheese
1 teaspoon fine sea salt
2 tablespoons olive oil
4 gluten-free burger buns (or milk buns if not gluten-free), halved
2 zucchini (courgettes), halved crossways then cut into thin slices lengthways
baby spinach leaves or rocket (arugula) leaves
Tomato and capsicum relish (page 18), to serve

Chop the garlic for **5 sec/speed 5**. Add the walnuts and chop for **3 sec/ speed 4**. Scrape down the side of the bowl. Add the beans, buckwheat flour, egg, basil, half the feta, salt and some freshly ground black pepper, to taste. Mix for **10 sec/speed 3** until well combined.

Preheat the grill (broiler) to high and line a baking tray with foil. Shape the mixture into four patties about 2.5 cm (1 in) thick.

Heat the oil in a large frying pan over medium heat. Cook the burgers for 3 minutes each side, or until golden. Meanwhile, toast the buns, cut side up, under the grill for 1–2 minutes. Remove and set aside.

Add the zucchini to the lined tray. Crumble over the remaining feta. Grill the zucchini for 5 minutes, or until the zucchini is tender and the feta is lightly golden.

Serve the burgers in the buns with the spinach, zucchini slices and some tomato and capsicum relish.

MAKE AHEAD: FREEZE
GLUTEN-FREE | VEGETARIAN

TIP

Make a double batch and freeze four uncooked patties. They keep for up to 6 months, just be sure to pop baking paper between them before wrapping up so they don't stick together. Freeze in an airtight bag or container.

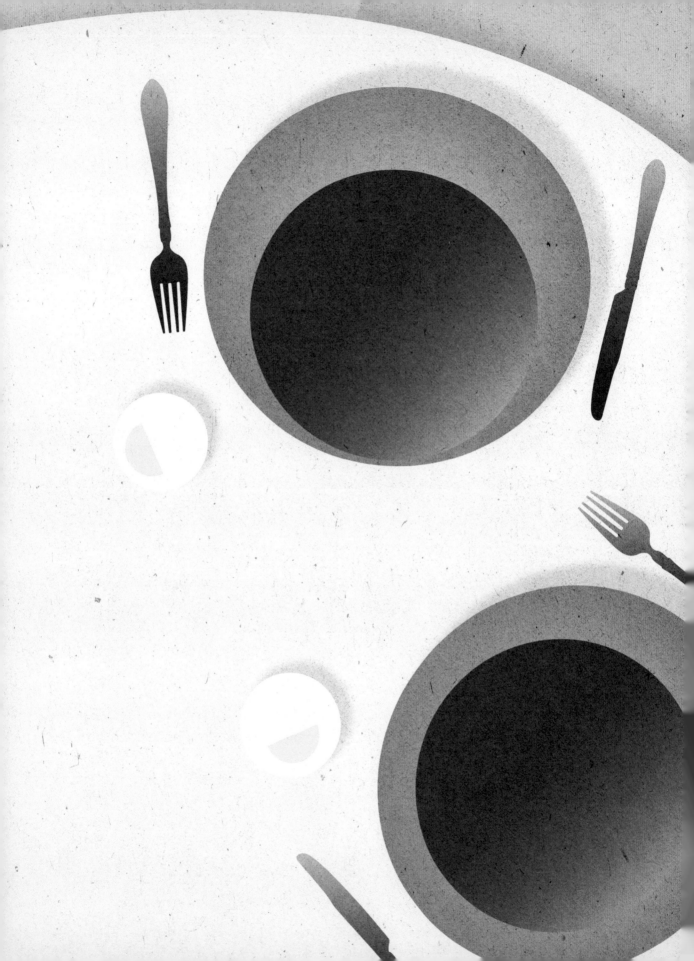

SLOWER DINNERS

MASTER STOCK CHICKEN

Master stocks can live a long life, developing over many years in some cases. But this version fast-tracks that first luscious, complex mouthful of broth. This keeps well in the freezer for up to 3 months.

SERVES 4

Preparation time 10 minutes + standing time
Cooking time 30 minutes

2 garlic cloves
2.5 cm (1 in) piece of ginger, peeled
1.5 litres (52 fl oz/6 cups) Chicken stock (page 31)
100 ml (3½ fl oz) light soy sauce
3 tablespoons Chinese rice wine (see Note)
125 ml (4 fl oz/½ cup) rice syrup or 4 tablespoons raw sugar
2 star anise
1 cinnamon stick
3 teaspoons Chinese five-spice
2 x 250 g (9 oz) chicken breasts
400 g (14 oz) Chinese broccoli
200 g (7 oz) broccolini, cut into 5 cm (2 in) lengths
600 g (1 lb 5 oz) fresh thin egg noodles, cooked according to packet instructions
sesame oil, to serve

Chop the garlic and ginger for **5 sec/speed 5**. Scrape down the side of the bowl. Add the stock, soy sauce, rice wine, rice syrup and dried spices. Cook for **15 min/90°C/speed 1**.

Meanwhile, add the chicken to the simmering basket, the broccoli and broccolini stems to the steaming basket and the leaves and florets to the steaming tray. Once the stock has been cooking for 15 minutes, carefully insert the simmering basket into the mixer bowl. Attach the steaming basket and tray to the mixer bowl lid. Cook for **15 min/ steam mode/speed 2**, or until the chicken is cooked through.

Set the chicken aside for 5 minutes to rest before slicing. Skim and discard any fat from the surface of the stock, then strain through a fine-mesh sieve lined with muslin (cheesecloth) or paper towel.

Serve the chicken with the noodles, broth and greens and a drizzle of sesame oil.

DAIRY-FREE

NOTE

Chinese rice wine is called shaoxing wine, and it's available in selected supermarkets and Asian food stores.

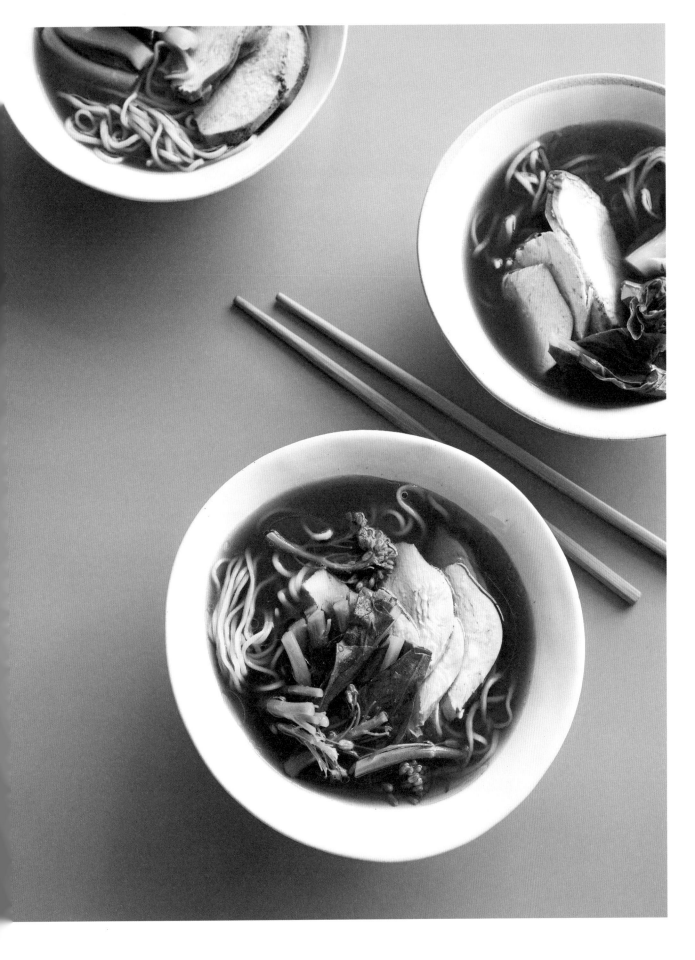

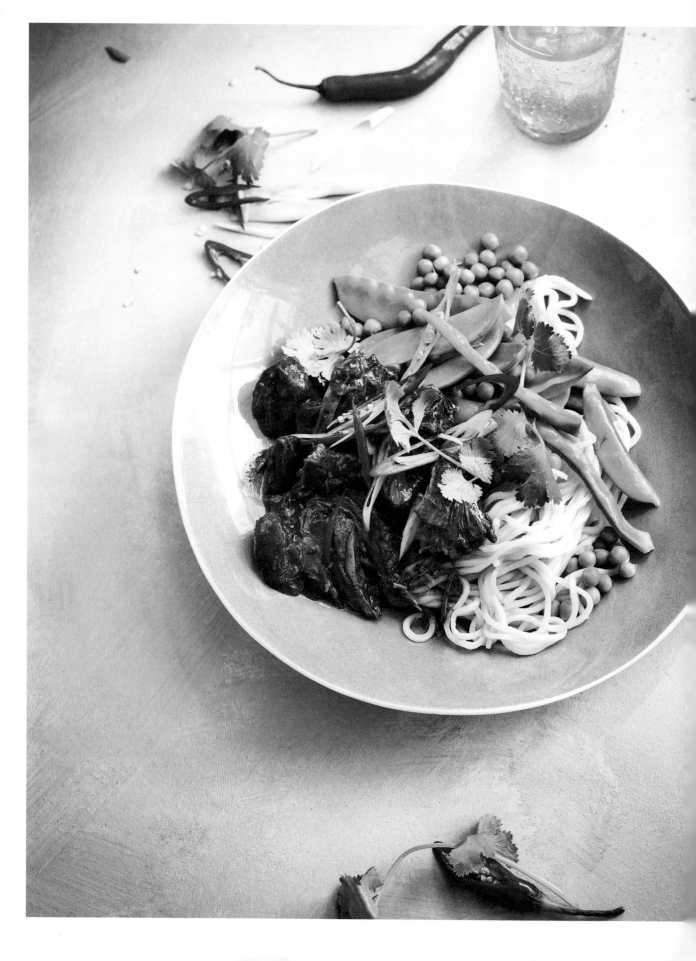

FIVE-SPICED BEEF

Slower-cooked dinners, like this, present a great opportunity to batch cook. The secondary and cheaper cuts of meat used for slow-cooking are packed with flavour, and will keep for up to 3 months if frozen in an airtight container (see Tip).

SERVES 4
Preparation time 15 minutes + standing time
Cooking time 2 hours

Five-spiced beef
3 teaspoons Chinese five-spice
2 tablespoons cornflour
   (cornstarch)
600 g (1 lb 5 oz) chuck steak,
   trimmed and cut into
   4 cm (1½ in) pieces
20 g (¾ oz) dried shiitake
   mushrooms, soaked in 600 ml
   (21 fl oz) boiling water for
   at least 10 minutes
1 tablespoon coconut oil or
   grapeseed oil

3 tablespoons kecap manis
   (see Note)

Veggies and noodles
200 g (7 oz) each of sugar snap
   peas and snow peas (mangetout),
   trimmed, strings removed
150 g (5½ oz) frozen green peas
600 g (1 lb 5 oz) fresh noodles
optional toppings: thinly sliced long
   red chilli, coriander (cilantro)
   sprigs and shredded spring onion
   (scallion), to serve

Combine the five-spice powder and cornflour in a bowl and season with sea salt. Toss the beef in this mixture until well coated. Drain the soaked mushrooms, reserving their soaking liquid. Remove and discard their stems, then halve or quarter the caps.

Put the coconut oil, beef, any remaining cornflour mixture, mushrooms and their soaking liquid, and the kecap manis into the mixer bowl. Cook for **105 min/110°C/reverse stir/soft stir**.

Once the time is up for the beef, add the sugar snap peas to the steaming basket and the snow peas and frozen peas to the steaming tray. Carefully remove the measuring cup and attach the steaming basket to the mixer bowl lid. Cook for **12 min/steam mode/reverse stir/soft stir**, or until the vegetables are tender.

Prepare the noodles according to the packet instructions, then serve the beef with the noodles, vegetables and your choice of toppings.

MAKE AHEAD: FREEZE
DAIRY-FREE | NUT-FREE

TIP

If freezing, skip the steps to make the veggies and noodles until you are reheating the beef.

NOTE

Kecap manis is a dark, sweet syrupy Indonesian soy sauce, available in Asian supermarkets.

CHICKEN AND HALOUMI PIDE

A pide is a Turkish pizza but don't let that fool you, the dough can also be used for a traditional Italian pizza simply by swapping the toppings.

SERVES 4

Preparation time 40 minutes + standing time
Cooking time 30 minutes

Pide toppings
200 g (7 oz) haloumi cheese
250 g (9 oz) minced (ground)
    chicken
2 tablespoons extra virgin olive oil
3 tablespoons Za'atar (page 42)
150 g (5½ oz) baby spinach leaves
250 g (9 oz) cherry tomatoes, halved
1 egg, lightly beaten
lemon wedges, to serve

Dough
375 g (13 oz/2½) cups plain
    (all-purpose) flour
1 teaspoon fine sea salt
1 x 7 g (⅙ oz) sachet instant dried
    yeast
1 teaspoon raw, white or
    caster (superfine) sugar
250 g (9 oz) water

Mix all of the dough ingredients together for **10 sec/speed 1**. Knead for **3 min/dough mode**. Transfer to a greased bowl, cover with a tea towel and set aside in a warm draught-free place for 1 hour, or until the dough doubles in size.

Meanwhile, grate the haloumi for **6 sec/speed 9**. Transfer to a bowl. (Don't rinse the mixer bowl.) Add the chicken, oil and 2 tablespoons of za'atar. Cook for **5 min/120°C/speed 1**. Add the spinach and cook for **2 min/120°C/speed 1**. Transfer the mixture to a sieve and drain any excess liquid. Set aside to cool. Once cool, mix in half of the grated haloumi.

Preheat the oven to 230°C (450°F) and line two large baking trays with baking paper. Punch down the dough and cut it in half. Shape one of the halves into an oval-shaped ball. Then, using a rolling pin or your hands, roll or stretch the dough out to a long oval shape about 35 x 18 cm (14 x 7 in). Transfer this to one of the lined trays, then repeat with the other half.

Divide the chicken mixture evenly between the bases, leaving a 2.5 cm (1 in) border around the edges. Top with the tomatoes, then scatter over the remaining haloumi and the za'atar. Fold the dough over to partially cover the filling and crimp the edges between your fingertips, pressing down firmly. Lightly brush the edges with the beaten egg to coat. Bake in the oven for 15–20 minutes until golden and cooked, swapping the trays halfway through. Serve with lemon wedges.

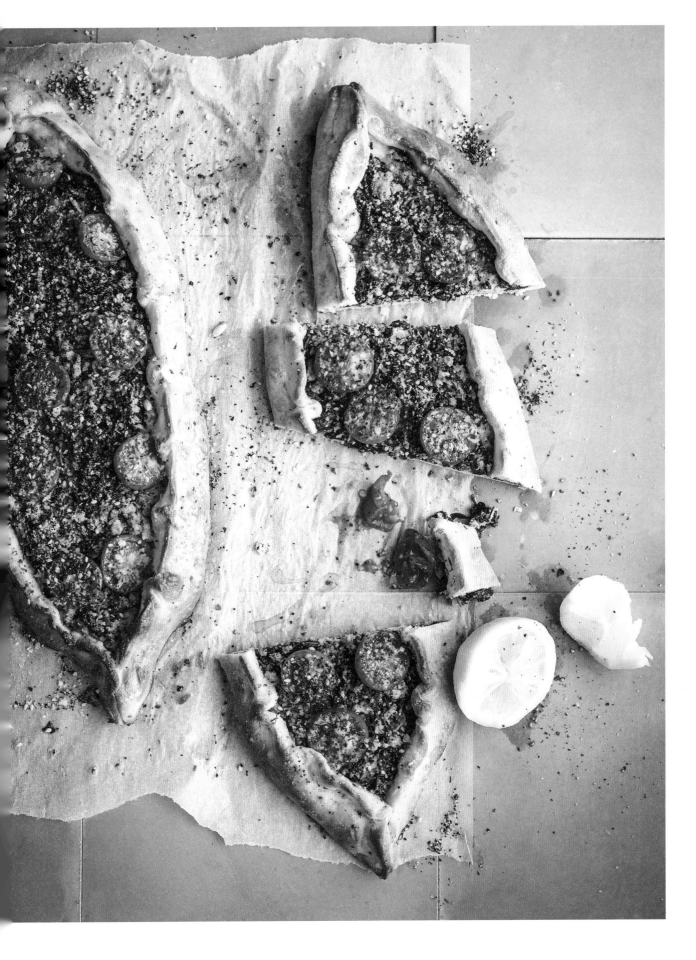

MEXICAN PULLED PORK

Pulled pork is a special treat in our house, especially when it's served with pineapple – it's one of those classic combinations that always goes down well. Chipotle chillies in adobo sauce are spicy, so it's best to add them to taste. You can find them in tins in gourmet food stores. Pulled pork can be served in many ways, but my favourite is piled on top of baked corn tortilla chips (aka healthier nachos). It's also great with a jacket potato. Just when you thought your mixer couldn't possibly perform another task, it pulls the pork for you! It's well worth making a double batch and storing one of them in an airtight container in the freezer for up to 3 months.

SERVES 4
Preparation time 10 minutes
Cooking time 1 hour 30 minutes

1 red onion, peeled and quartered
3 garlic cloves
150 g (5½ oz) sweet pineapple, coarsely chopped
1–2 chipotle chillies in adobo sauce
¼ teaspoon ground cloves
2 teaspoons cumin seeds, toasted
2 teaspoons dried oregano
3 tablespoons white vinegar
200 g (7 oz) Naked pasta sauce (page 14) or tinned chopped tomatoes
600 g (1 lb 5 oz) pork shoulder, trimmed of any fat and cut into 6 cm
    (2½ in) pieces
corn tortillas, to serve
optional for serving: lime wedges and a few slices of charred pineapple

Chop the onion and garlic for **5 sec/speed 5**. Scrape down the side of the bowl. Add the remaining ingredients, except for the pork and serving and season with sea salt. Blend for **20 sec/speed 6**. Scrape down the side of the bowl.

Add the pork and cook for **90 min/100°C/reverse stir/speed 1**, or until tender and 'pulled'.

Serve the pork with tortillas, some lime wedges for squeezing over and a few slices of charred pineapple.

MAKE AHEAD: FREEZE
DAIRY-FREE | GLUTEN-FREE | NUT-FREE

LAMB IN MINT SAUCE

Now this is one of those timeless family classics, but even better because it's all made in one dish! Less washing up! The main ingredient in mint sauce is normally sugar, but here I've used apples, carrots and peas for some natural sweetness.

SERVES 4

Preparation time 10 minutes
Cooking time 1 hour 20 minutes

1 leek, white part only, roughly chopped
2 garlic cloves
600 g (1 lb 5 oz) green apples, quartered and cored
125 ml (4 fl oz/½ cup) apple cider or white wine vinegar
2 large handfuls mint leaves
3 teaspoons raw sugar or 1 tablespoon maple syrup
500 g (1 lb 2 oz) lamb shoulder, cut into 5 cm (2 in) pieces
3 carrots, peeled and cut into bite-sized pieces
500 g (1 lb 2 oz) waxy potatoes, peeled and cut into bite-sized pieces
300 g (10½ oz) frozen peas, thawed

Blend the leek, garlic, apples, vinegar, half a handful of mint leaves and the sugar for **30 sec/speed 7**.

Add the lamb to the mixer bowl and season well with sea salt and pepper. Add the carrots to the steaming basket and the potatoes to the steaming tray. Attach the steaming basket and tray, instead of the measuring cup, to the mixer bowl lid. Cook for **75 min/100°C/ reverse stir/soft stir**, or until the lamb is tender.

Meanwhile, finely chop the remaining mint leaves.

Once the lamb has been cooking for 75 minutes, add the remaining mint to the mixer bowl and the peas to the steaming basket and cook for a further **5 min/100°C/reverse stir/soft stir**.

Serve the lamb and mint sauce with the steamed vegetables.

DAIRY-FREE | GLUTEN-FREE | NUT-FREE

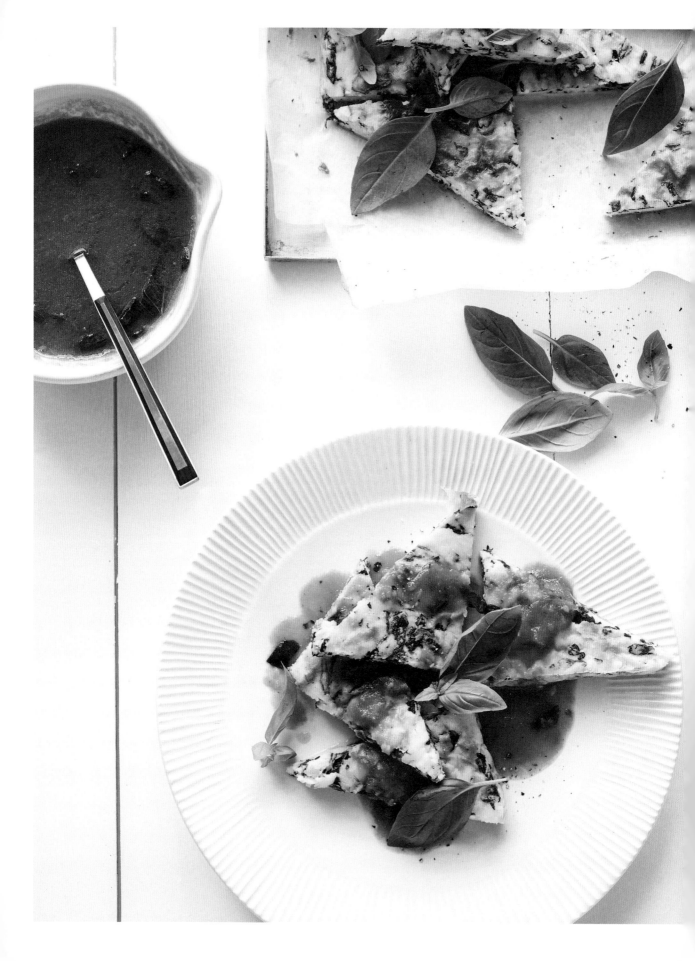

SPINACH AND RICOTTA TRIANGLES

This is my cheat's version of semolina and ricotta gnocchi or gnudi. It's much easier to pour the mixture straight into a tray and cut it into whichever shapes you like best.

SERVES 4

Preparation time 20 minutes + standing time
Cooking time 45 minutes

50 g (1¾ oz) parmesan cheese, roughly chopped, plus extra, grated (see Note on page 36)
150 g (5½ oz) fine semolina
2 tablespoons extra virgin olive oil, plus extra to serve
200 g (7 oz) baby spinach leaves
375 g (13 oz) fresh ricotta cheese

2 eggs
1 large handful basil leaves, plus extra to serve
400 g (14 oz) Naked pasta sauce (page 14) or tinned chopped tomatoes
pine nuts or slivered almonds, toasted, to serve (optional)

Preheat the oven to 180°C (350°F). Line a 30 x 20 cm (12 x 8 in) baking tin with enough baking paper to overhang, so you can lift out the bake. Grate the parmesan for **15 sec/speed 10**. Transfer to a small bowl.

Add 250 g (9 oz) of water to the mixer bowl, season with sea salt and bring to the boil for **5 min/100°C/speed 1**. Gradually pour in the semolina, then add 1 tablespoon of the oil and cook for **3 min/95°C/speed 3**.

Meanwhile, add the spinach to a large heatproof bowl and cover with boiling water. Set aside for 20 seconds, or until wilted. Drain in a sieve under cold running water until cool, then place in a clean tea towel and squeeze out as much excess liquid as possible. Add the spinach and ricotta to the mixer bowl. Blend for **10 sec/speed 5**. Add half of the parmesan and the eggs, then season with salt and pepper. Mix for **30 sec/speed 3**. Transfer the mixture to the lined tin and evenly distribute around the tin. Bake in the oven for 20–25 minutes until lightly golden and firm. Remove and set aside for 5 minutes.

Add the basil leaves, pasta sauce and remaining oil to the washed mixer bowl. Season to taste. Cook for **10 min/95°C/speed 1**.

Carefully, lift out the ricotta bake from the baking tin and move to a chopping board. Cut into triangles then serve with the pasta sauce, remaining parmesan, basil leaves, pine nuts and extra virgin olive oil.

MAKE AHEAD: FREEZE
VEGETARIAN

TIP

If you are making a batch of these to freeze, remove them from the oven after 20 minutes, when the surface is lightly golden and the mixture is firm to the touch. You can either slice and reheat in the oven or pan-fry. They make really great snacks for the kids too.

MOROCCAN LAMB AND APRICOT STEW

The tartness of the dried apricots really makes this dish — their flavour goes so well with the full flavour of the lamb and all of those veggies. The harissa isn't too hot, but feel free to leave it out if you prefer. If you intend to freeze this, I suggest adding the apricots and veggies after thawing and reheating. But it will still be good, either way.

SERVES 4

Preparation time 15 minutes
Cooking time 1 hour 25 minutes

2 cm (¾ in) piece of ginger, peeled
1 red onion, peeled and quartered
1 large handful coriander (cilantro), stems roughly chopped, leaves reserved
1 tablespoon ras el hanout spice mix
1 tablespoon olive oil
600 g (1 lb 5 oz) lamb shoulder, cut into 4 cm (1½ in) pieces
400 g (14 oz) Naked pasta sauce (page 14) or tinned chopped tomatoes
1 tablespoon harissa paste (optional)
75 g (2¾ oz) dried apricots, halved
300 g (10½ oz) cauliflower, cut into large florets
500 g (1 lb 2 oz) peeled pumpkin (winter squash), cut into 4 cm (1½ in) pieces
couscous (or quinoa, for a gluten-free option), to serve
blanched almonds, toasted, to serve

Chop the ginger, onion, coriander stems and ras el hanout together for **5 sec/speed 5**. Scrape down the side of the bowl. Add the oil and cook for **3 min/120°C/speed 1**.

Add the lamb, pasta sauce and the harissa, if using, and season with sea salt. Cook for **60 min/100°C/reverse stir/soft stir**.

Add the apricots, cauliflower and pumpkin. Cook for **20 min/100°C/ reverse stir/soft stir**, or until the lamb and vegetables are tender. Season to taste with sea salt and pepper.

Meanwhile, prepare the couscous according to the packet instructions. Serve the stew with couscous and scatter over the coriander leaves and almonds.

MAKE AHEAD: FREEZE
DAIRY-FREE

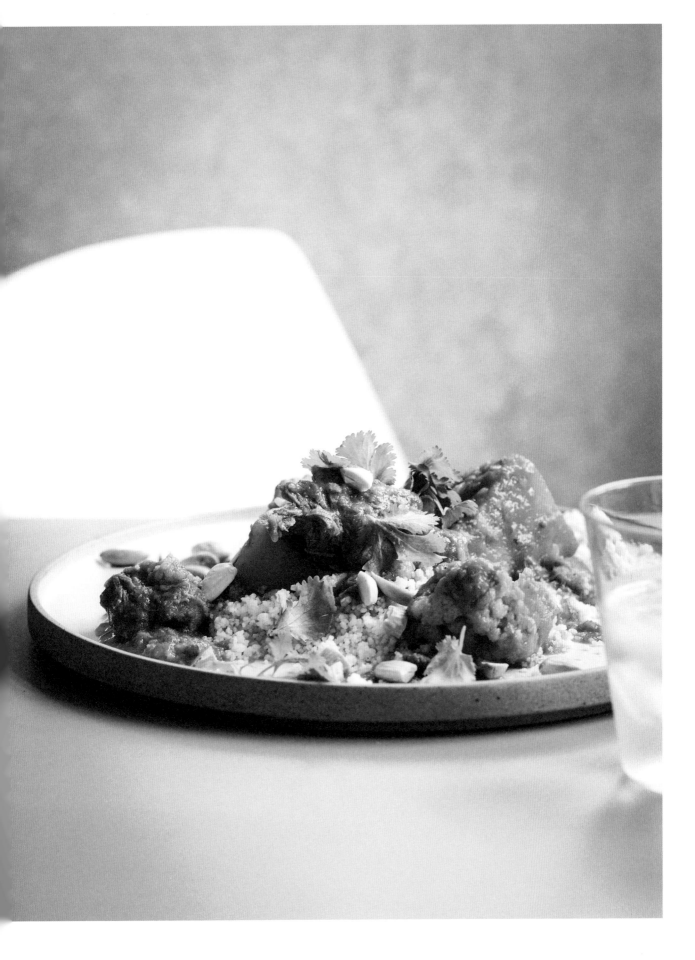

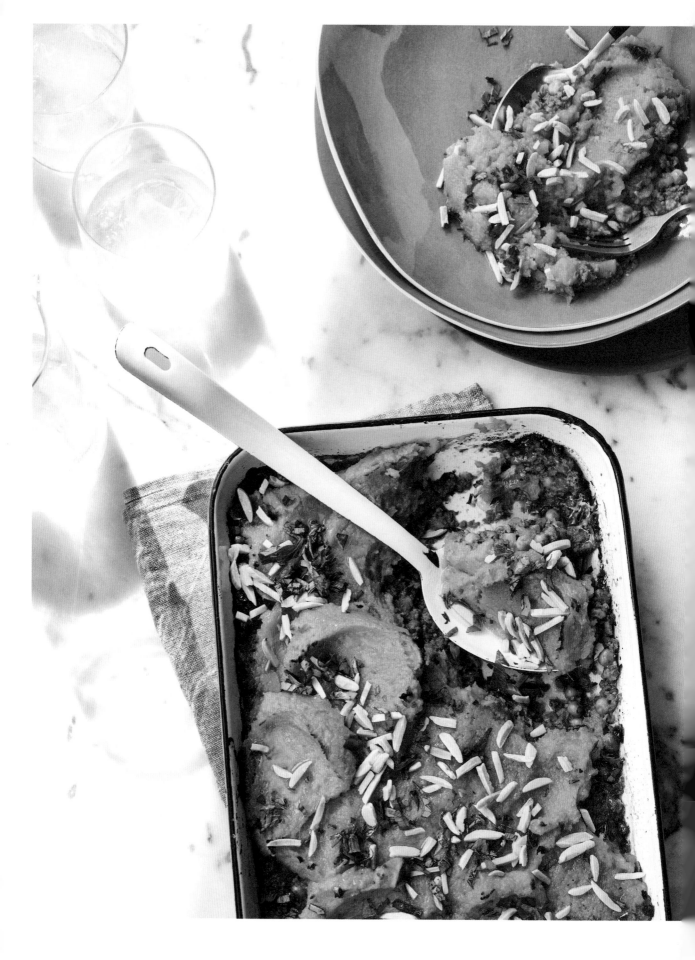

VEGGIE-PACKED SHEPHERD'S PIE

Win the kids over with this comforting pie. Toasted nuts on top instead of breadcrumbs give this an amazing gluten-free crunch, and if you omit the butter, this is also dairy-free.

SERVES 4

Preparation time 15 minutes
Cooking time 35 minutes

1 red onion, peeled and quartered
2 carrots, peeled and roughly chopped
2 celery stalks, roughly chopped
3 tablespoons olive oil
500 g (1 lb 2 oz) lean minced (ground) lamb
2 tablespoons cornflour (cornstarch) or gluten-free plain flour
125 ml (4 fl oz/½ cup) Chicken or Vegetable stock (pages 31 and 32)
125 g (4½ oz/½ cup) Naked pasta sauce (page 14) or
   tinned chopped tomatoes
2 tablespoons worcestershire sauce
200 g (7 oz) frozen peas
4 tablespoons roughly chopped parsley
800 g (1 lb 12 oz) Root veg mash (page 42)
30 g (1 oz) Butter (page 22), chopped
slivered almonds, toasted, to serve (optional)

Chop the onion, carrot and celery for **3 sec/speed 5**. Scrape down the side of the bowl. Add 1 tablespoon of oil and cook for **3 min/120°C/speed 2**. Add the lamb to the bowl and season well with sea salt and pepper. Cook for **5 min/120°C/speed 1**.

Meanwhile, whisk the cornflour in a large jug with a small amount of stock until smooth. Whisk in the remaining stock, pasta sauce and worcestershire sauce. Add this stock mixture to the mixer bowl and cook for **20 min/120°C/reverse stir/speed 1**. Add the peas and half the parsley and mix for **20 sec/speed 2**. Season to taste with sea salt and pepper, then transfer to a 2–2.5 litre (70–87 fl oz/8–10 cup) pie dish.

Preheat the oven grill (broiler) to high. Spread the mash evenly over the filling to cover. Dot over the butter then place the pie under the grill for 5 minutes. Once the pie is lightly golden and the butter has melted, serve with the remaining parsley and toasted almonds scattered on top.

MAKE AHEAD: FREEZE
GLUTEN-FREE

GREEK-STYLE LAMB WITH FETA, DILL AND LEMON

One of my favourite ways to cook meat in my mixer is in a really flavourful vegetable purée. Here, the capsicum and garlic blend provides a really nice background for the other Mediterranean flavours. This lamb is another great recipe for freezing, and can be enjoyed loads of other ways: served with rice, in pita bread, or used as a filling in a filo pastry pie. Your device should be able to accommodate a double batch of this, so it's well worth cooking once for twice the reward.

SERVES 4

Preparation time 15 minutes
Cooking time 1 hour 20 minutes

2 red capsicums (peppers), stems and seeds removed, roughly chopped
4 garlic cloves
500 g (1 lb 2 oz) boned lamb shoulder or leg, cut into 4 cm (1½ in) pieces
2 tablespoons finely chopped rosemary
2 tablespoons red wine vinegar
1 teaspoon sugar
120 g (4¼ oz) feta cheese
2 Lebanese (short) cucumbers, roughly chopped
250 g (9 oz) cherry tomatoes, quartered
pita breads or flatbreads, to serve

Blend the capsicums and garlic for **20 sec/speed 7**. Scrape down the side of the bowl. Add the lamb, rosemary, vinegar and sugar and season with salt and pepper. Cook for **80 min/100°C/reverse stir/soft stir**, or until tender.

Serve the lamb in the sauce with the feta crumbled on top next to the chopped cucumbers, cherry tomatoes and pita bread.

MAKE AHEAD: FREEZE
NUT-FREE

FISH SAN CHOY BAU

I admit this isn't a likely suspect in a slower-cooked chapter, but it's such an easy way to 'cook' fresh fish without actually doing any cooking at all. San choy bau is one of those family favourites that goes way back. I love the way it brings everyone together around the table, each person can help themselves and dig in! No cutlery required.

You can add all sorts of fillings to the lettuce cups, but I especially love the combination here. I love making this in the summer months – turning that morning's fresh fish into a light supper to be enjoyed on a balmy evening. I like to use different coloured capsicums for a variation of colour, but it's not essential.

SERVES 4

Preparation time 20 minutes + standing time

2 x 250 g (9 oz) fish fillets (1 salmon and 1 firm white fish, such as ling), cut into 1 cm (½ in) pieces (see Note)
1 corn cob, kernels removed
juice of 1 lime
juice of 1 lemon
2 vine-ripened tomatoes, quartered, seeds removed and discarded
1 Lebanese (short) cucumber, halved lengthways, seeds removed, roughly chopped
2 capsicums (peppers), stems and seeds removed, roughly chopped
1 x 270 ml (9½ fl oz) tin coconut cream
1 ripe avocado, stone removed, peeled and cut into 1 cm (½ in) pieces
2 tablespoons finely chopped chives
2 baby cos lettuces, trimmed, leaves separated

Combine the fish, corn, and lime and lemon juices in a large, non-metallic bowl and season with salt and pepper. Cover with plastic wrap and refrigerate for at least 1 hour, or even overnight.

In two batches, chop the tomatoes, cucumber and capsicums for **2 sec/speed 4**. Transfer the vegetable mixture, coconut cream, avocado and chives to the bowl with the fish and mix until well combined.

Serve the san choy bau with the lettuce leaves.

MAKE AHEAD: FRIDGE
DAIRY-FREE | GLUTEN-FREE | NUT-FREE | LOW-CARB

TIP

You want the freshest of fresh fish when making this. Frozen won't do. I suggest visiting a fishmonger's and asking them for the freshest fillets they have.

THE CLEVEREST MEATLOAF

Meat may not be the sole ingredient in this meatloaf, but once cooked, there are no signs of anything *but* meat! Veggie-phobes won't know what hit them. (Hence, the name.) You can freeze an uncooked loaf for up to 3 months as long as it's well wrapped and protected from the freezer. Delicious with a generous spoonful of the Root veg mash on page 42 and some warmed Tomato and capsicum relish (page 18).

SERVES 6

Preparation time 15 minutes
Cooking time 50 minutes

olive oil, to grease
50 g (1¾ oz) parmesan cheese, roughly chopped
1 red onion, peeled and quartered
2 garlic cloves
2 carrots, peeled and coarsely grated
2 zucchini (courgettes), coarsely grated
1 x 400 g (14 oz) tin kidney beans, rinsed and drained
2 tablespoons fresh oregano or 3 teaspoons dried oregano
105 g (3¾ oz/1 cup) instant oats
500 g (1 lb 2 oz) minced (ground) beef
2 eggs
3 teaspoons fine sea salt

Preheat the oven to 180°C (350°F) and grease and line a 1.5–2 litre (52–70 fl oz/6–8 cup) loaf (bar) tin with baking paper. Grate the parmesan for **15 sec/speed 10**. Add the onion, garlic, carrot and zucchini. Chop for **5 sec/speed 5**. Add the kidney beans and oregano. Chop for **5 sec/speed 5**. Scrape down the side of the bowl.

Insert the whisk attachment and add the oats, beef, eggs, salt and some pepper. Mix for **2 min/speed 2** until well combined. Transfer this mixture into the prepared tin and spread it out evenly using a large spoon. Ensure there are no air pockets. Bake in the oven for 50 minutes, or until cooked through. Allow the meatloaf to stand for 10 minutes before turning it out and slicing.

Serve the meatloaf with some warmed relish and generous spoonfuls of mash.

MAKE AHEAD: FREEZE
NUT-FREE

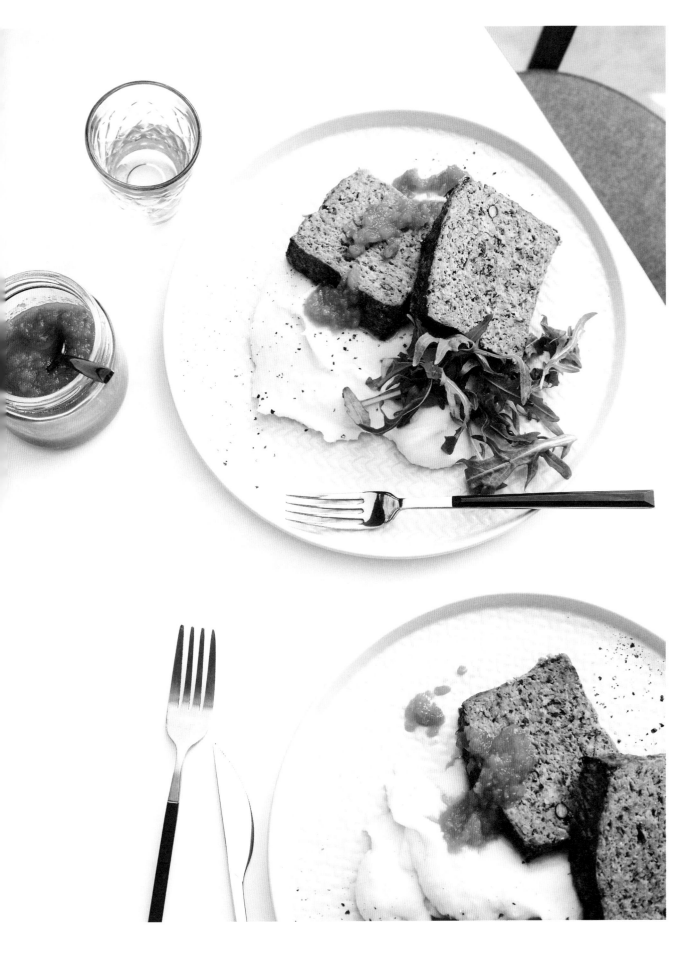

LENTIL AND MUSHROOM MOUSSAKA

If you're looking for a vegetarian hit – one to please veggos and omnivores equally – this is the recipe for you. If the ricotta you buy is firm (the style normally found in a large wheel), then you'll only need 1 egg. However, if it's from a tub and of a much softer consistency, then it's best to add 2 eggs. You can freeze this moussaka for up to 3 months and finish cooking it in the oven at a later date. And, if you're part of a resolutely meat-eating household, you can also make this into a meat feast by using the Lamb bolognese (page 116) or lasagne meat filling (page 160) in place of the lentil base.

SERVES 4

Preparation time 30 minutes
Cooking time 35 minutes

50 g (1¾ oz) parmesan cheese, roughly chopped (see Note on page 36)
1 red onion, peeled and quartered
400 g (14 oz) Swiss brown mushrooms, brushed clean
2 tablespoons oregano leaves
2 tablespoons extra virgin olive oil, plus extra for brushing
2 teaspoons ground cinnamon
140 g (5 oz/¾ cup) dried French green lentils, rinsed and drained
400 g (14 oz) Naked pasta sauce (page 14) or tinned chopped tomatoes
500 g (1 lb 2 oz) eggplant (aubergine), thinly sliced into 5 mm (¼ in) slices
375 g (13 oz) fresh ricotta cheese
1–2 eggs (see recipe intro), lightly beaten
flat-leaf (Italian) parsley leaves, roughly chopped, to serve
rocket (arugula) leaves, roughly chopped to serve

Grate the parmesan for **15 sec/speed 10**. Transfer to a bowl and set aside. Chop the onion, mushrooms and oregano for **5 sec/speed 4**. Scrape down the side of the bowl. Add 1 tablespoon of the oil and the cinnamon, and cook for **3 min/120°C/speed 2**.

Meanwhile, preheat the oven to 200°C (400°F) and grease a 1.5 litre (52 fl oz/6 cup) dish. Add the lentils, pasta sauce and 250 g (9 oz/1 cup) of water to the mixer bowl. Add the large pieces of eggplant in a single layer to the steaming basket and the remainder to the steaming tray. Attach the steaming basket and tray, instead of the measuring cup, to the mixer bowl lid.

Cook for **15 min/steam mode/reverse stir/speed 1** until the eggplant is tender. Remove the steaming basket and tray and carefully insert the measuring cup into the lid. Continue to cook the lentil mixture for **10 min/100°C/reverse stir/speed 1** until the lentils are just tender.

Meanwhile, combine the ricotta, half the parmesan and the beaten egg in a bowl. Season with salt and pepper. Line the base of the dish with some of the steamed eggplant slices.

Transfer the lentil mixture to the dish and smooth over the surface. Arrange a single layer of eggplant slices on top of the lentil mixture. Pour over the ricotta mixture and smooth it over the surface to cover evenly. Scatter oven the remaining parmesan.

Bake in the oven for 5 minutes, then switch the oven onto grill (broiler) mode on high. Grill for 5 minutes, or until the moussaka is turning golden in parts.

Remove and set aside for 5–10 minutes before serving.

Serve scattered with the chopped parsley and rocket leaves.

MAKE AHEAD: FREEZE
GLUTEN-FREE | NUT-FREE | PALEO | VEGETARIAN | LOW-CARB

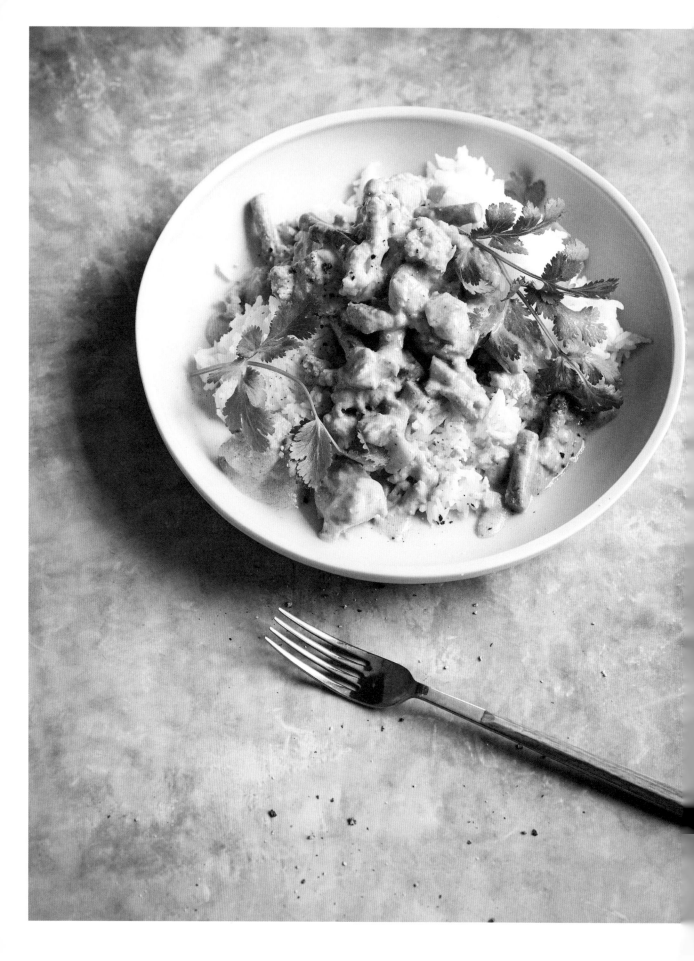

SATAY CHICKEN CURRY

Using homemade nutter butter and tahini is very satisfying in this curry, plus it means no nasty ingredients sneak in under the radar. But any good-quality nut butter will be fine. If you prefer the cauliflower broken down a little more to disguise it, add it at the same time as the chicken. Curry powders come in varying strengths, so refer to the back of the packet to determine how much to use. Once cooked, you can keep this in an airtight container in the freezer for up to 3 months.

SERVES 4

Preparation time 20 minutes
Cooking time 25 minutes

2 carrots, peeled and roughly chopped
500 g (1 lb 2 oz) chicken thighs, trimmed, cut into
    3 cm (1¼ in) pieces
3–4 tablespoons Malaysian curry powder
1 tablespoon coconut or other neutral oil
2 teaspoons fine sea salt
400 ml (14 fl oz) tin coconut milk
4 tablespoons Nutter butter (page 21)
2 tablespoons Tahini (page 39)
350 g (12 oz) cauliflower, cut into small florets
150 g (5½ oz) green beans, trimmed and cut into 2 cm lengths
2 tablespoons each rice syrup, lime juice and tamari (gluten-free soy sauce)
optional serving ingredients: steamed rice or Cauliflower rice (page 158),
    a few sprigs of coriander (cilantro) and Gomasio (page 39) (optional)

Chop the carrot for **2 sec/speed 5**. Scrape down the side of the bowl.

Add the chicken, curry powder, oil and salt. Cook for **5 min/120°C/ reverse stir/speed 1**. Add the coconut milk, nutter butter, tahini and 4 tablespoons of water. Cook for **5 min/100°C/reverse stir/speed 1**.

Add the cauliflower and cook for **5 min/100°C/reverse stir/soft stir**.

Add the beans and cook for **5 min/100°C/reverse stir/soft stir**.

Add the rice syrup, lime juice and tamari. Cook for **1 min/100°C/speed 1**.

Serve the curry with steamed rice or cauliflower rice, and top with a few coriander sprigs and a sprinkle of gomasio.

MAKE AHEAD: FREEZE
DAIRY-FREE | GLUTEN-FREE

VEGETARIAN CHILLI

I like using black-eyed peas because, unlike a lot of other pulses, you can throw them into your mixer with other ingredients without having to cook them first. It's important not to season the chilli with any salt until *after* the beans are cooked, otherwise they will remain firm and take much longer to cook. If you have the time and the inclination, you can easily make sour cream to serve with this by mixing labne with some lime juice. You can serve this chilli in a number of ways: with roasted sweet potatoes, steamed rice or tortillas. Fussy eaters have no excuse! Any leftovers can be stored in an airtight container in the freezer for up to 6 months.

SERVES 4

Preparation time 10 minutes + standing time
Cooking time 50 minutes

2 red capsicums (peppers), stems and seeds removed, roughly chopped
1 leek, white part only, roughly chopped or
    1 red onion, peeled, quartered and roughly chopped
2 garlic cloves
2 teaspoons ground cumin
2 large handfuls coriander (cilantro), leaves and stems, roughly chopped
1–2 chipotle chillies in adobo sauce (these are spicy, so add to your taste)
2 corn cobs, kernels removed
220 g (7¾ oz/1 cup) dried black-eyed peas, soaked in water overnight, rinsed and drained
500 g (1 lb 2 oz) Naked pasta sauce (page 14) or 400 g (14 oz) tinned chopped tomatoes with 100 ml (3½ fl oz) water
serving options: jacket potatoes, feta cheese or Labne (page 27) and some lime wedges

Chop the capsicum, leek, garlic, cumin, coriander stems and the chipotle for **5 sec/speed 4**. Scrape down the side of the bowl. Add the corn, peas and pasta sauce. Cook for **50 min/100°C/reverse stir/soft stir** until the peas are tender. Season to taste with sea salt.

Spoon the chilli over a jacket potato, crumble over some feta or add a spoonful of labne and serve with lime wedges.

MAKE AHEAD: FREEZE
GLUTEN-FREE | NUT-FREE | VEGETARIAN

BEEF AND BLACK-EYED PEA CHILLI

A versatile chilli recipe is a great thing to have up your sleeve, and this one fits the bill. It can be made with other cuts of beef, such as gravy beef (shin), brisket or even cheeks. And, like so many of the recipes in this chapter, it freezes really well and keeps for up to 3 months, so it's a great one to batch cook.

SERVES 4

Preparation time 15 minutes + standing time
Cooking time 1 hour 55 minutes

1 red capsicum (pepper), stem and seeds removed, roughly chopped
1 onion, peeled and quartered
2 garlic cloves
1 tablespoon olive oil
2 teaspoons ground cumin
2 teaspoons smoked paprika
1 teaspoon ground chilli
1 teaspoon dried oregano
500 g (1 lb 2 oz) chuck steak, trimmed and cut into 2.5 cm (1 in) cubes
2 fresh or dried bay leaves
400 g (14 oz) Naked pasta sauce (page 14) or tinned chopped tomatoes
150 g (5½ oz/¾ cup) black-eyed peas, soaked in water overnight, rinsed and drained
serving options: steamed rice and lime wedges (optional)

Chop the capsicum, onion and garlic for **4 sec/speed 5**. Scrape down the side of the bowl. Add the oil, spices and the oregano, then cook for **3 min/120°C/speed 1**.

Add the beef, bay leaves and pasta sauce. Cook for **60 min/120°C/ reverse stir/soft stir**.

Add the black-eyed peas and cook for a further **50 min/95°C/ reverse stir/soft stir** until tender. Season to taste with sea salt.

Serve the chilli with steamed rice and some lime wedges, if desired.

MAKE AHEAD: FREEZE
DAIRY-FREE | GLUTEN-FREE | NUT-FREE

BUTTER CHICKEN WITH CAULIFLOWER RICE

A mild curry everyone can enjoy is always a winner, and this one uses yoghurt instead of cream, so it's better for you. Cauliflower rice is a great way to up that veggie goodness.

SERVES 4

Preparation time 10 minutes + standing time
Cooking time 20 minutes

4 cm (1½ in) ginger, peeled and roughly chopped
2 tablespoons garam masala
2–3 long red chillies, roughly chopped (taste for heat then add accordingly)
1 teaspoon fine sea salt
200 g (7 oz/¾ cup) Homemade yoghurt (page 26)
600 g (1 lb 5 oz) chicken thighs, trimmed and cut into 3 cm (1¼ in) pieces
60 g (2¼ oz) cashews or blanched almonds
1 red onion, peeled and roughly chopped
50 g (1¾ oz) Butter (page 22)
400 g (14 oz) Naked pasta sauce (page 14) or tinned chopped tomatoes
3 tablespoons tomato paste (concentrated purée)
1–2 tablespoons lime juice
mint or coriander (cilantro) leaves, to serve

Cauliflower rice
750 g (1 lb 10 oz) cauliflower, roughly chopped

Blend the ginger, garam masala, chillies and salt for **20 sec/speed 7**. Scrape down the side of the bowl. Add the yoghurt and mix for **10 sec/speed 3**. Transfer to a bowl, add the chicken pieces and mix to coat well. Marinate in the fridge for at least 30 minutes, or preferably overnight.

In two batches, chop the cauliflower for **5 sec/speed 6**. Transfer to the steaming basket. Rinse out the mixer bowl, then chop the cashews for **10 sec/speed 7**. Add the onion and chop for **5 sec/speed 5**. Scrape down the side of the bowl. Add the butter and cook for **3 min/120°C/speed 1**.

Add the pasta sauce and tomato paste and blend for **20 sec/speed 7**. Scrape down the side of the bowl. Add the chicken, all of the marinade and the lime juice. Attach the steaming basket to the mixer bowl lid and cook for **15 min/steam mode/reverse stir/speed 1**. Serve the curry with the cauliflower rice and mint leaves.

MAKE AHEAD: FREEZE
GLUTEN-FREE

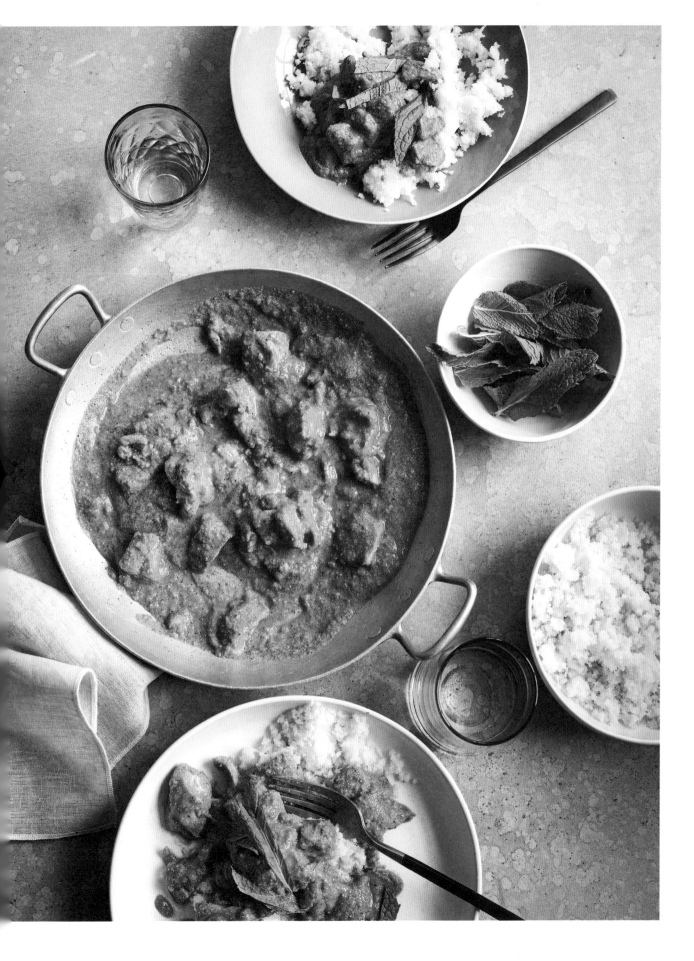

FAMILY LASAGNE

Lasagne is one of those dishes I find difficult to say no to — that second (or even third) helping is just sort of inevitable. Cauliflower bechamel really lightens up this classic, while sneakily adding in a good amount of another vegetable.

SERVES 4–6

Preparation time 30 minutes
Cooking time 1 hour 20 minutes

25 g (1 oz) parmesan cheese, roughly chopped
2 leeks, white part only, roughly chopped
2 carrots, peeled and roughly chopped
2 celery stalks, roughly chopped
1 tablespoon extra virgin olive oil, plus extra to serve
500 g (1 lb 2 oz) mixture of minced (ground) beef and pork, or just beef mince
400 g (14 oz) Naked pasta sauce (page 14) or tinned chopped tomatoes
4 tablespoons tomato paste (concentrated purée)
2 fresh or dried bay leaves
3 tablespoons fresh oregano or basil leaves
250 g (9 oz) lasagne sheets
1 quantity Cauliflower bechamel (page 36)

Grate the parmesan for **15 sec/speed 10**. Transfer to a bowl and set aside. Chop the leek for **8 sec/speed 5**, then transfer to a bowl. Chop the carrot and celery for **5 sec/speed 5**. Return the leek to the mixer bowl and scrape down the side. Add the oil and cook for **3 min/120°C/speed 1**.

Add the meat, pasta sauce, tomato paste and herbs. Season well with sea salt and pepper. Cook for **45 min/100°C/reverse stir/speed 1**.

Preheat the oven to 190°C (375°F). Spoon a thin layer of bechamel onto the base of a 2.5–3 litre (87–105 fl oz/10–12 cup) baking dish. Layer with lasagne sheets to cover, then evenly layer in half of the meat mixture followed by one-third of the remaining bechamel. Repeat the layering again: lasagne sheets, meat, bechamel, then finish with one more layer of lasagne sheets and the remaining bechamel. Scatter over the parmesan to cover.

Bake the lasagne in the oven for approximately 30 minutes or until golden and cooked (use the cooking time on the pasta packet as a guide).

MAKE AHEAD: FREEZE
NUT-FREE

TIPS

There are many different lasagne sheets available, like instant cook or gluten-free. Use the cooking time on the packet as a guide to how long you should bake it in the oven.

To freeze, wrap the uncooked lasagne (in its baking dish) really well then store in the freezer for up to 3 months.

VEGETARIAN LASAGNE

I've used meaty mushrooms here in exactly the same way as I would beef in a classic lasagne. Everybody loves it!

SERVES 4–6
Preparation time 30 minutes
Cooking time 50 minutes

25 g (1 oz) parmesan cheese, chopped (see Note on page 36)
500 g (1 lb 2 oz) mixed mushrooms such as cup, shiitake and button
1 red capsicum (pepper), stem and seeds removed, roughly chopped
200 g (7 oz) Naked pasta sauce (page 14) or tinned chopped tomatoes
1 red onion, peeled and quartered
1 carrot, peeled and roughly chopped

1 celery stalk, roughly chopped
2 tablespoons extra virgin olive oil
1 large handful basil leaves
¼ teaspoon dried chilli flakes
4 tablespoons tomato paste (concentrated purée)
200 g (7 oz) baby spinach leaves
250 g (9 oz) lasagne sheets
1 quantity Cauliflower bechamel (page 36)

Grate the parmesan for **15 sec/speed 10**. Transfer to a small bowl. In two batches, chop the mushrooms for **3 sec/speed 4**. Transfer to a bowl. Chop the capsicum for **5 sec/speed 5**. Scrape down the side of the bowl. Add the pasta sauce and blend for **15 sec/speed 8**. Transfer to a bowl. Chop the onion, carrot and celery for **5 sec/speed 5**. Add the oil and season with sea salt and pepper. Cook for **3 min/120°C/speed 1**.

Preheat the oven to 190°C (375°F). Add the mushrooms to the mixer with the pasta sauce mixture, half the basil, the chilli flakes and tomato paste. Cook for **15 min/100°C/reverse stir/speed 2**. Transfer to a large bowl. Add the spinach, remaining basil and season with sea salt and pepper, mixing until the spinach wilts.

Spoon a thin layer of bechamel onto the base of a 2.5–3 litre (87–105 fl oz/10–12 cup) baking dish. Layer with lasagne sheets to cover, then evenly spread over half of the mushroom mixture, then one-third of the remaining bechamel. Continue layering: lasagne sheets, mushroom mixture then bechamel. Finish with another layer of lasagne sheets and top with the remaining bechamel. Scatter over the parmesan to cover. Bake for approximately 30 minutes, or until golden and cooked.

See photograph on pages 162–3.

MAKE AHEAD: FREEZE
NUT-FREE | VEGETARIAN

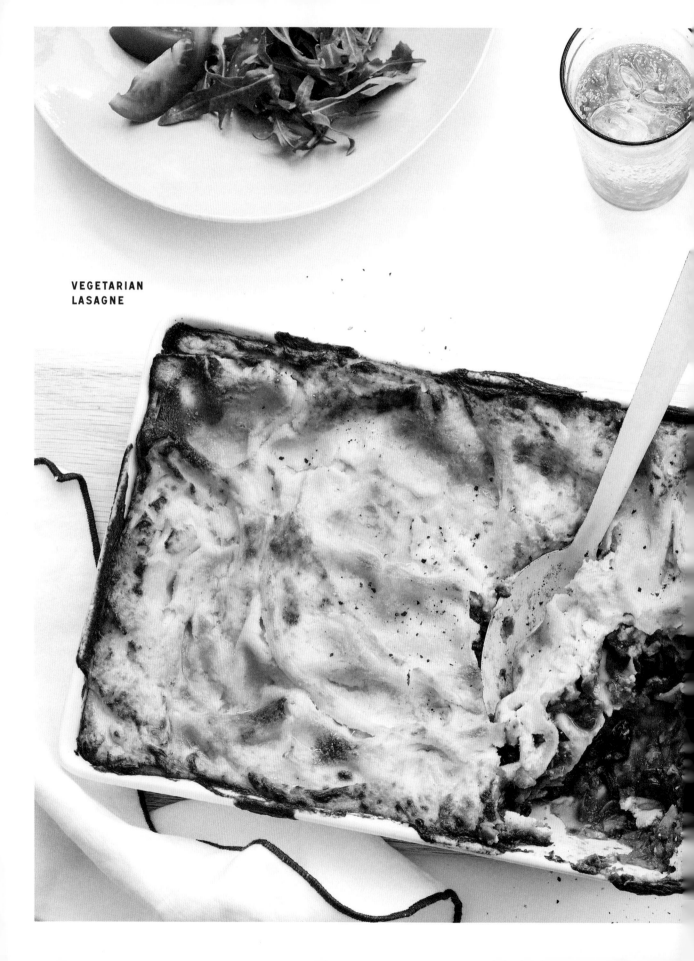

VEGETARIAN
LASAGNE

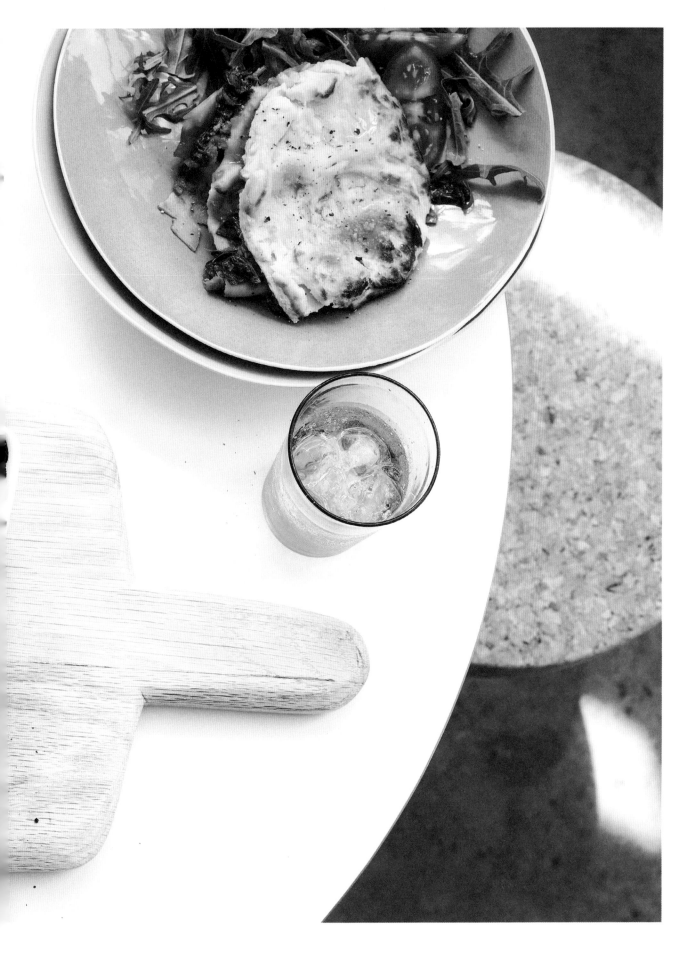

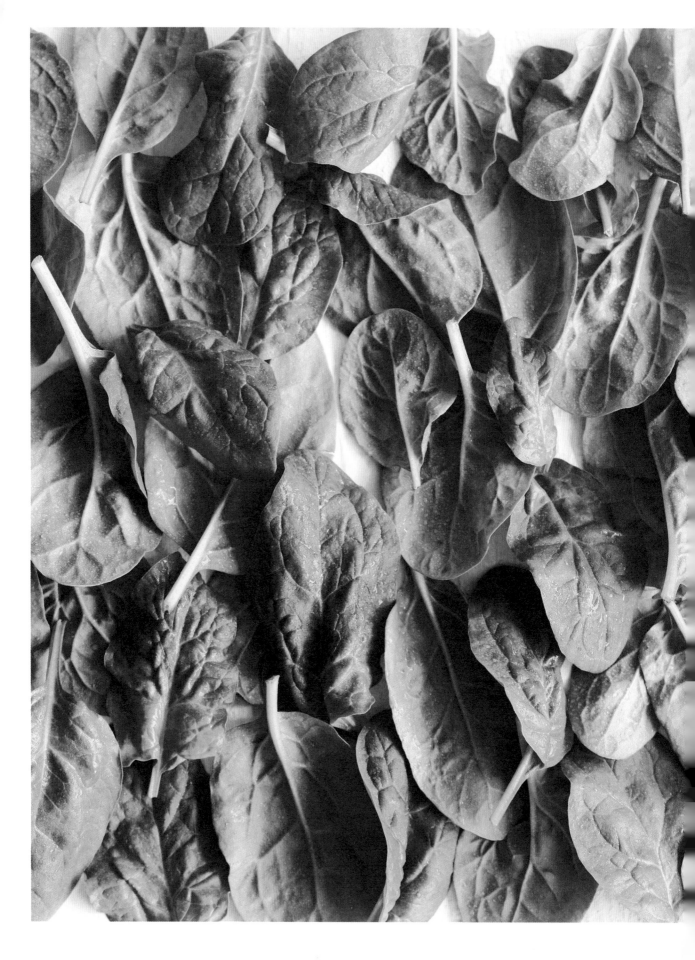

CHICKPEA AND SPINACH CURRY

What a delicious all-rounder this curry is, not to mention a great way to introduce Indian spices to the kids. Cover the chickpeas in enough water to remain completely submerged then soak them overnight before making this. This can be stored in an airtight container and kept in the freezer for up to 6 months.

SERVES 4

Preparation time 10 minutes + standing time
Cooking time 1 hour 5 minutes

2 garlic cloves
2.5 cm (1 in) piece of ginger, peeled
1 red onion, peeled and quartered
2 long green chillies, stems removed, 1 thinly sliced
½–1 teaspoon ground chilli (add to your taste)
1 teaspoon each ground turmeric and ground cumin
25 g (1 oz) Butter (page 22), see Tip
25 g (1 oz) coconut oil
200 g (7 oz/1 cup) dried chickpeas, soaked in water overnight, rinsed and drained
1 litre (35 fl oz/4 cups) Vegetable stock (page 32) or water
250 g (9 oz) baby spinach leaves
2 teaspoons fine sea salt
roti, to serve

Chop the garlic, ginger, onion and the whole chilli for **5 sec/speed 5**. Scrape down the side of the bowl. Add the dried spices, butter and coconut oil. Cook for **3 min/120°C/speed 1**.

Add the chickpeas and stock. Cook for **55 min/90°C/reverse stir/ speed 1**, or until the chickpeas are tender.

Add the spinach and salt and cook for **5 min/90°C/reverse stir/ speed 1**. Blend for **3 sec/speed 4**.

Serve the curry with the sliced chilli sprinkled on top and some warm roti.

MAKE AHEAD: FREEZE
GLUTEN-FREE | NUT-FREE | VEGETARIAN

TIP

A really easy way to make this recipe dairy-free and vegan is to swap butter for coconut oil.

BUTTERMILK HOT WINGS WITH CHIMICHURRI POTATO SALAD

Most families have a favourite hot sauce on hand. If using Tabasco, start off with 1 teaspoon as it's far more concentrated than other hot sauces. The longer you marinate these wings, the juicier and more delicious they'll be. Two days is ideal.

SERVES 4

Preparation time 10 minutes + standing time
Cooking time 35 minutes

250 ml (9 fl oz/1 cup) Buttermilk
  (page 22)
3–4 tablespoons hot sauce
1 kg (2 lb 4 oz) chicken wings
800 g (1 lb 12 oz) waxy, red-skinned
  potatoes, washed, halved and
  sliced into 1 cm (½ in) pieces

4 tablespoons Chimichurri
  (page 44)
165 g (5¾ fl oz/⅔ cup) Mayonnaise
  (page 47)
2 Lebanese (short) cucumbers,
  roughly chopped
2 celery stalks, roughly chopped

Mix the buttermilk and hot sauce in an airtight container large enough to fit the wings. Toss the wings in the marinade until well combined. Marinate in the fridge for at least 1 hour, preferably longer (or freeze for up to 6 months and thaw out in the fridge a day before cooking).

Preheat the oven to 200°C (400°F). Tip the chicken wings and their marinade into a large baking dish, then arrange them in a single layer.

Add 500 g (1 lb 2 oz) of water to the mixer bowl. Place the larger pieces of potato in the steaming basket and put the smaller pieces on the steaming tray, ensuring the steam can pass through. Attach the steaming basket and tray to the mixer bowl lid. Cook for **25 min/ steam mode/speed 3** until tender.

Meanwhile, bake the wings for 35 minutes, or until golden and cooked through. Combine the chimichurri and mayonnaise in a large bowl. Add the potatoes, cucumbers and celery and toss well. Season with salt and pepper then serve the wings with the potato salad.

MAKE AHEAD: FRIDGE | FREEZER
GLUTEN-FREE | NUT-FREE

TIP
If you want to, you can line the large baking dish with baking paper before the chicken goes in. It makes washing up that little bit easier.

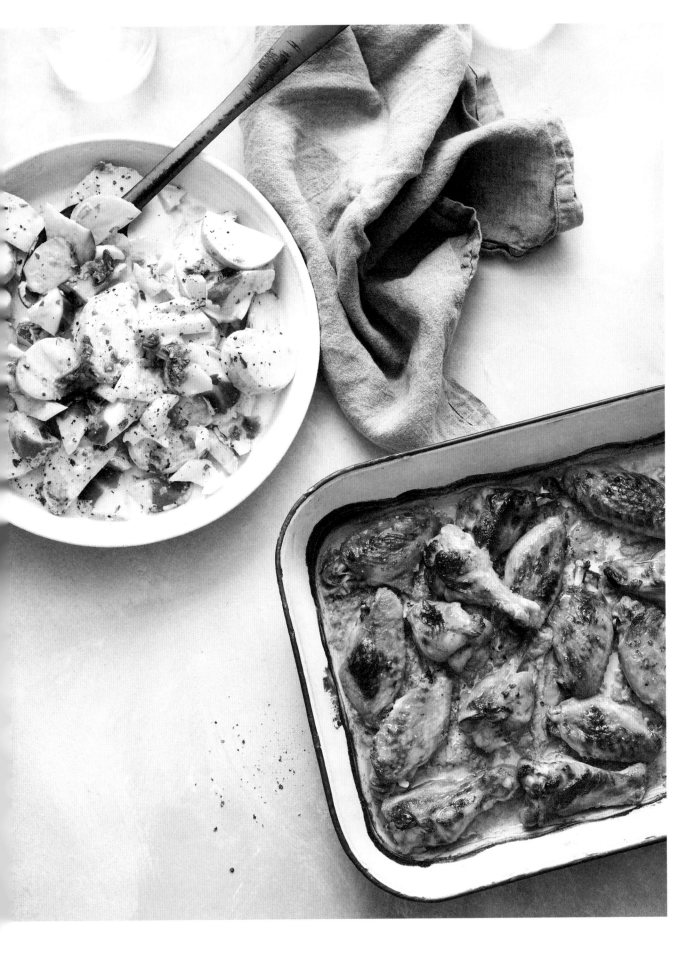

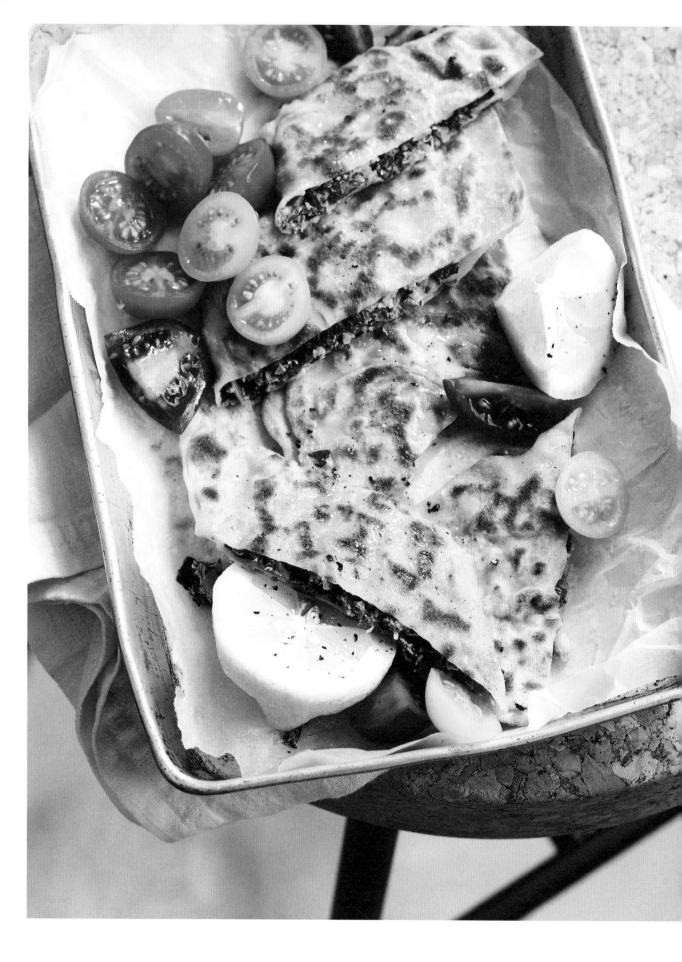

SPINACH AND CHEESE GOZLEME

Turkish gozlemes from outdoor food stalls are always pretty good, but I often wish they had more filling. Making your own is a fun way to entertain the kids on a lazy weekend – let them roll out the dough and add all the fillings. Leave the dough overnight, if you can, then use it up right away.

SERVES 4
Preparation time 45 minutes + standing time
Cooking time 25 minutes

375 g (13 oz/2½ cups) plain (all-purpose) flour, plus extra to dust
1 teaspoon fine sea salt
olive oil, for greasing
400 g (14 oz) silverbeet (Swiss chard), leaves finely shredded, stems chopped
250 g (9 oz) English spinach, thinly sliced
3 tablespoons finely chopped mint or dill
200 g (7 oz) fresh ricotta cheese
200 g (7 oz) feta cheese
1 egg
400 g (14 oz) mixed cherry tomatoes, halved
lemon wedges, to serve

Mix the flour, salt and 250 g (9 oz) of water for **10 sec/speed 1**. Scrape down the side of the bowl. Knead for **5 min/dough mode**. Transfer to a greased bowl, cover with a tea towel and set aside for at least 6 hours.

Combine the silverbeet leaves, spinach and mint in a large bowl. Chop the silverbeet stems for **4 sec/speed 5** then add to the silverbeet mixture. Blend the ricotta, feta and egg in the mixer bowl for **10 sec/speed 3** until combined. Transfer to the bowl with the silverbeet mixture and mix well.

Preheat the oven to 120°C (235°F). Divide the dough into six and wrap five portions in plastic wrap. On a lightly floured surface, roll the unwrapped portion of dough into a 3 mm (⅛ in) thick round. Place one-sixth of the silverbeet filling on one half of the circle. Fold over the uncovered half, pressing down the edges firmly to seal. Repeat with the remaining dough and filling. Grease the base of a large frying pan or hot plate with oil and heat over medium heat. Cook two gozleme at a time for 6–8 minutes, turning often, until golden and cooked. Keep the cooked gozleme warm in the oven while you cook the rest. Serve with chopped tomatoes and lemon wedges.

NUT-FREE | VEGETARIAN

FALAFEL WITH LEMON TAHINI DRESSING

Falafel are one of the best vegetarian go-to meals. You can buy them pre-made, but making your own takes them to a whole new level. Believe me, it is worth the effort. You can make a double batch, and freeze half for up to 6 months in an airtight container. You can shape them before freezing, or just freeze the mixture. Whatever is easiest! Just keep in mind that they will expand because of the baking powder, so best to make them on the smaller side. The dressing can also be made ahead and kept in the fridge for up to 2 weeks. These go really well with the cucumber tabbouleh on page 108 (minus the salmon). When frying, remember a quick cook is a good cook, as you want them to be nice and fluffy. Take care not to put too many of them in the pan at one time otherwise they will lower the temperature of the oil and take too long to cook.

SERVES 4–6

Preparation time 25 minutes + standing time
Cooking time 15 minutes

Falafel
300 g (10½ oz/1½ cups) dried chickpeas
3 garlic cloves
1 onion, peeled and roughly chopped
30 g (1 oz) coriander (cilantro), including the stems, roughly chopped,
    plus extra sprigs to serve
50 g (1¾ oz) parsley, including the stems, roughly chopped,
    plus extra leaves to serve
1½ teaspoons baking powder
50 g (1¾ oz) sesame seeds
1 tablespoon Za'atar (page 42) or ground cumin
2 teaspoons fine sea salt
neutral oil, for shallow frying
flatbreads and chopped salad ingredients of your choice, to serve

Lemon tahini dressing
2 tablespoons lemon juice
3 tablespoons Tahini (page 39)
1½ tablespoons extra virgin olive oil

Cover the chickpeas completely in water, ensuring there is enough water to allow for the chickpeas to expand and still remain submerged. Leave to soak overnight, then rinse and drain well.

Chop the chickpeas, garlic, onion, coriander and parsley for **10 sec/speed 8**. Scrape down the side of the bowl and repeat the process. Add the baking powder, sesame seeds, za'atar and salt. Mix for **1 min/speed 3**. Roll the mixture into 3 cm (1¼ in) balls, then flatten slightly into discs and chill in the fridge for at least 15 minutes, or until needed. Preheat the oven to 120°C (235°F).

To make the dressing, blend all of the dressing ingredients with 3 tablespoons of water in the cleaned mixer bowl for **15 sec/speed 5**. Season to taste with sea salt. Transfer to a bowl and set aside.

Pour enough oil into a large, deep frying pan to come up 1.5 cm (⅝ in) up the side of the pan. Place over medium heat and bring to 170°C (340°F). If you don't have a thermometer, test the temperature of the oil by dropping a cube of bread into the oil. It should turn golden in 20 seconds. In batches, cook the falafel for 1–2 minutes on each side until golden and cooked. Remove and drain well on paper towel. Keep the cooked batches warm in the oven while you cook the remaining falafel.

Serve the falafel with flatbreads, chopped salad ingredients, a handful of herbs and the lemon tahini dressing.

See photograph on pages 172–3.

MAKE AHEAD: FREEZE
DAIRY-FREE | VEGAN

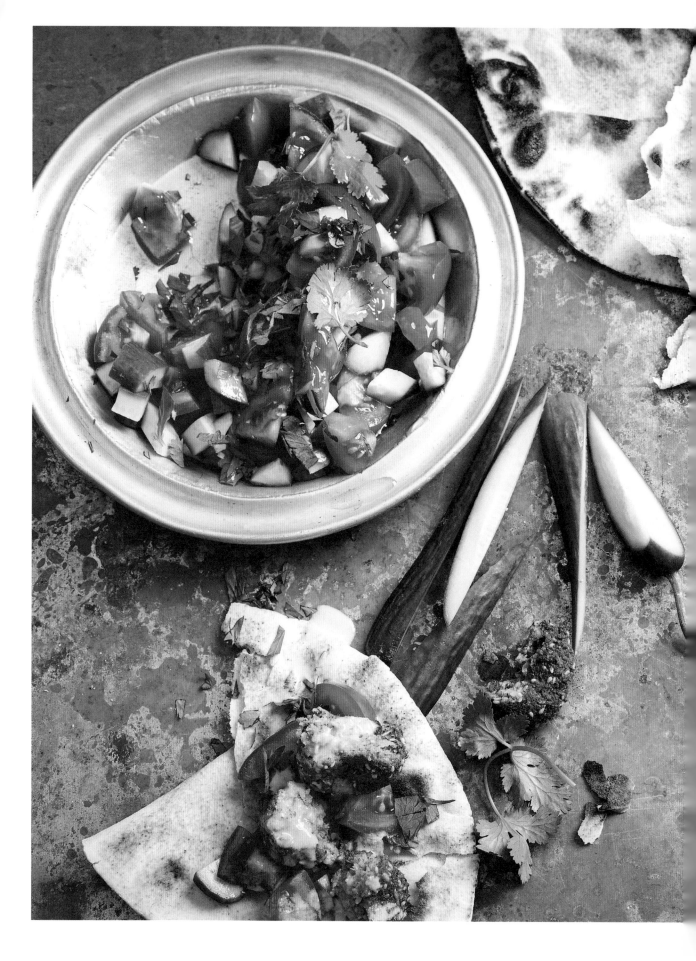

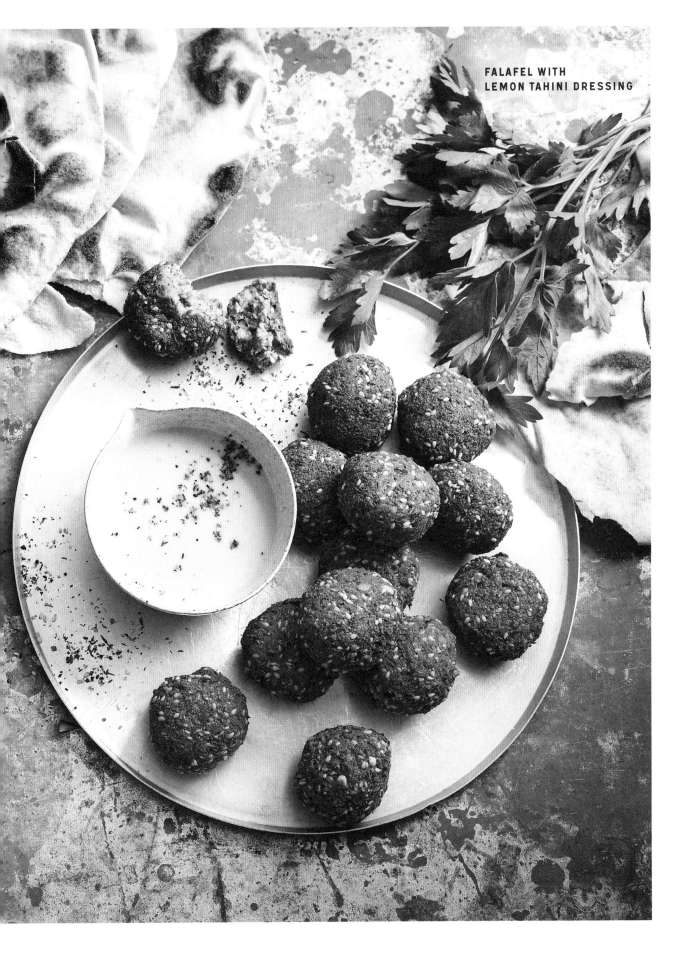

FALAFEL WITH
LEMON TAHINI DRESSING

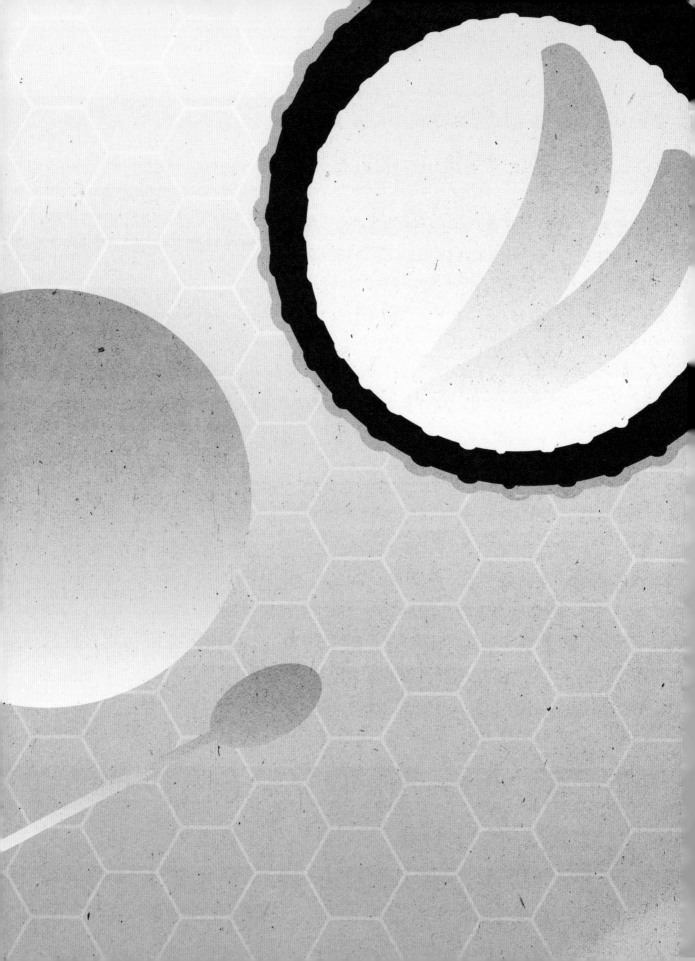

SWEET
SOMETHINGS

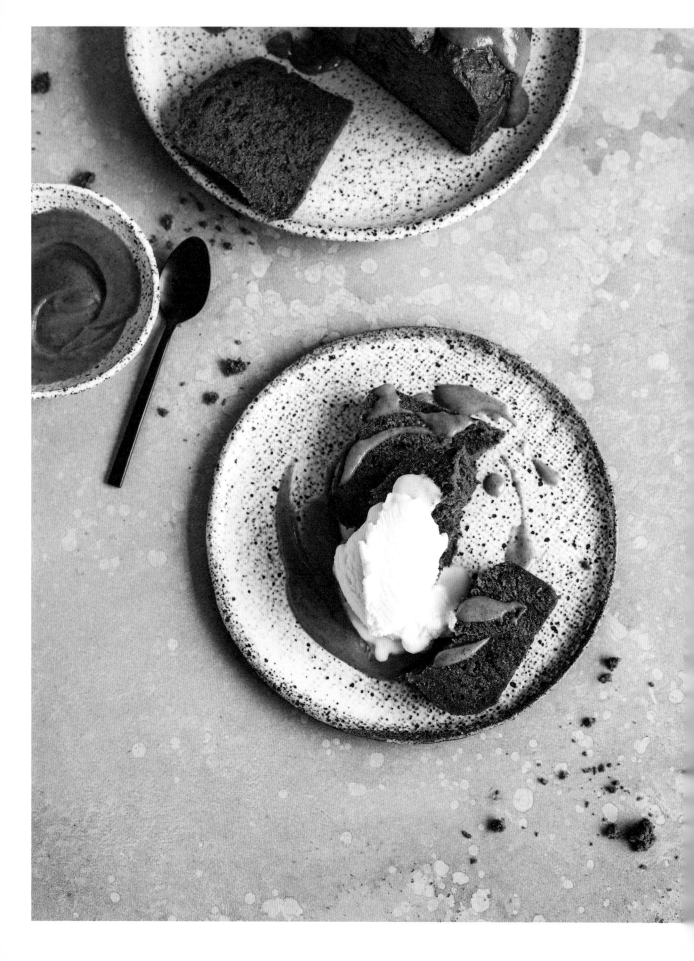

STEAMED DATE PUDDING WITH SALTED CARAMEL SAUCE

Just when you thought you couldn't get any more use out of your mixer, along comes this steamed dessert. It's easy to make and so comforting. A drizzle of salted caramel finishes things off perfectly.

SERVES 6

Preparation time 20 minutes + standing time
Cooking time 2 hours

200 g (7 oz) fresh pitted dates
200 g (7 oz/1 cup) pitted prunes
200 g (7 oz) Nutter butter (page 21)
125 ml (4 fl oz/½ cup) coconut oil
1 vanilla bean, split and seeds scraped, or
    1 teaspoon vanilla bean paste or extract
1½ teaspoons mixed spice
3 eggs
150 g (5½ oz/1 cup) self-raising flour
Vegan salted caramel sauce (page 51) and coconut sorbet (optional), to serve

NOTE

When steaming, it's important to keep the water temperature just below boiling point, otherwise the water will boil over and leach into the pudding. I place a heatproof bowl upside down over the lid to allow for the pudding to rise and expand.

TIP

You can make this up to a week in advance if you like, and keep it well-wrapped in the fridge. When you're ready to serve it, just steam in your mixer for 15 minutes to reheat. Easy.

Chop the dates and prunes for **4 sec/speed 5**. Scrape down the side of the bowl. Add the nutter butter, coconut oil, vanilla and mixed spice. Mix for **1 min/speed 3**. After 20 seconds, add one egg at a time until combined. Scrape down the side of the bowl.

Add the flour and mix for **1 min/dough mode**.

Line the simmering basket well with a large piece of baking paper with enough overhanging to cover the surface of the pudding. Transfer the pudding mixture to the lined simmering basket.

Add 500 g (1 lb 2 oz) of water to the mixer bowl and insert the simmering basket. Cook for **120 min/95°C/speed 2**, checking the water level halfway through, adding more if needed (see Note).

Carefully remove the pudding from the mixer bowl and set aside to cool for 10 minutes before serving.

Serve the pudding warm with a generous drizzle of salted caramel sauce and a spoonful of coconut sorbet, if you like.

MAKE AHEAD: FRIDGE
VEGETARIAN

BUTTERMILK PANNA COTTA WITH STEWED RHUBARB

A creamy panna cotta is just too hard to resist, but when buttermilk and yoghurt are replacing the cream, there's no need to fight it, or feel guilty about giving it to the kids. If you're trying to get ahead, you can make these up to 2 days in advance and keep them covered in the fridge.

SERVES 4

Preparation time 10 minutes + standing time
Cooking time 20 minutes

Panna cotta
2 gelatine leaves, soaked in water
250 ml (9 fl oz/1 cup) Buttermilk (page 22)
260 g (9¼ fl oz/1 cup) Homemade yoghurt (page 26)
1 teaspoon vanilla bean paste or extract
4 tablespoons maple syrup or rice syrup or 3 tablespoons of sugar
  (any kind of sugar except brown, which will be too sweet)

Stewed rhubarb
250 g (9 oz) rhubarb, cut into 4 cm (1½ in) lengths
3 tablespoons maple syrup or rice syrup, or 2 tablespoons sugar
1 teaspoon vanilla bean paste or natural vanilla extract
2 star anise (optional)
a pinch of salt

Place the gelatine leaves in a bowl and cover completely with cold water. Soak for 5 minutes, or until softened. Put the buttermilk, yoghurt, vanilla, maple syrup and a pinch of sea salt into the mixer bowl. Cook for **5 min/75°C/speed 1**.

Squeeze out any excess liquid from the gelatine leaves then add them to the buttermilk mixture. Cook for **1 min/75°C/speed 2**.

Divide the mixture evenly between four 125 ml (4 fl oz/½ cup) ramekins or moulds. Cover each with plastic wrap then place in the refrigerator for at least 4 hours until set, but preferably overnight.

Put all of the ingredients for the rhubarb in the mixer bowl. Cook for **10 min/95°C/reverse stir/speed 1** until the rhubarb is tender. Serve the panna cotta with the hot or cold stewed rhubarb.

MAKE AHEAD: FRIDGE
GLUTEN-FREE | NUT-FREE | VEGETARIAN

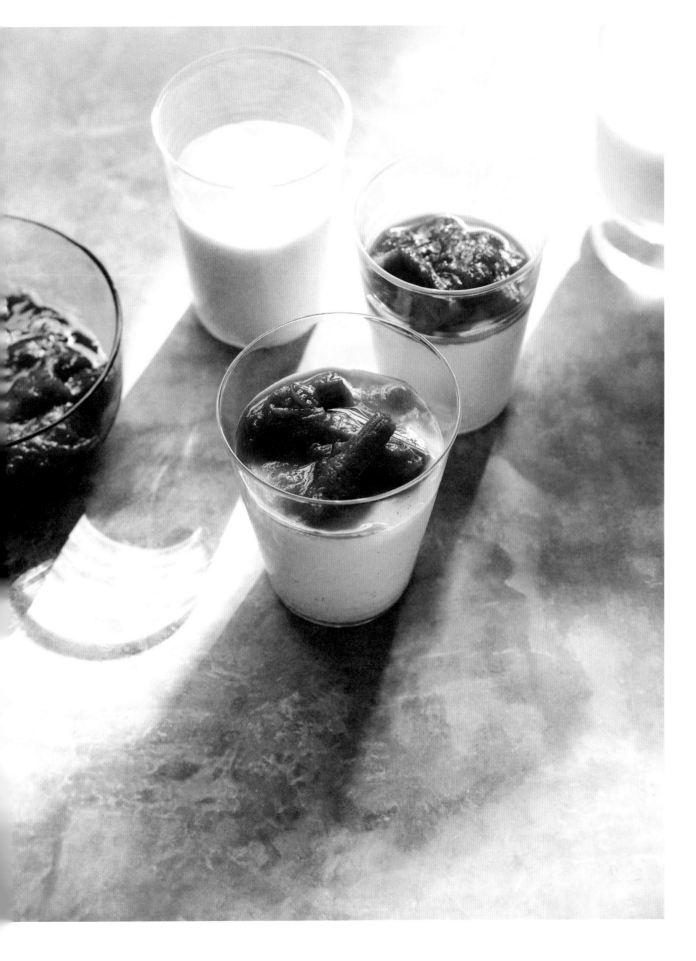

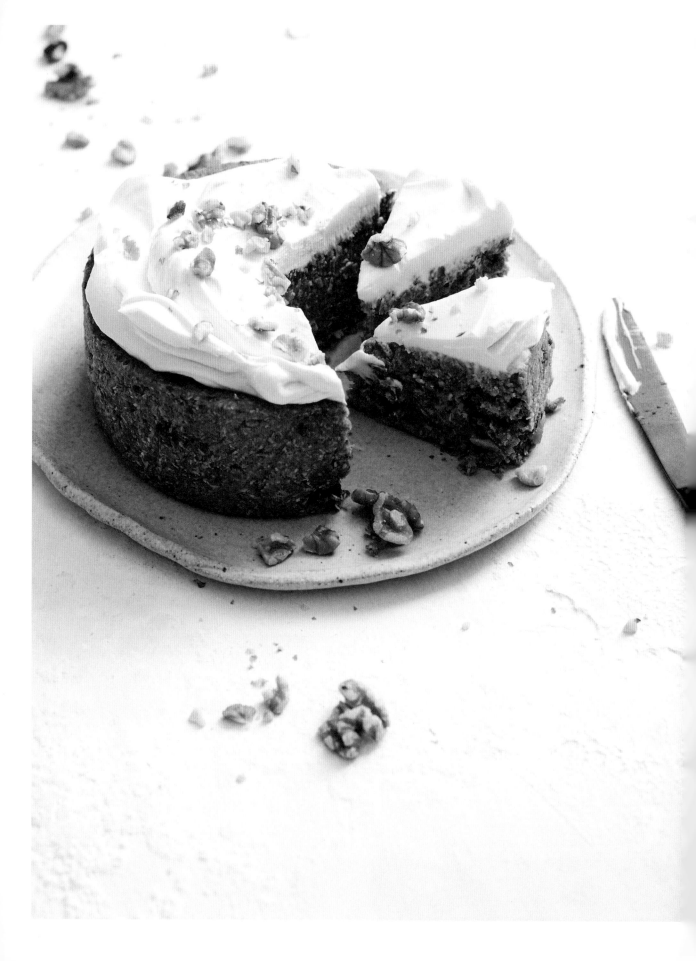

NO-BAKE CARROT CAKE

This is the easiest cake because you don't even need to turn on the oven. I often get looks of confusion when I tell people that it's entirely raw. Not only does it taste that good, but the texture is surprisingly similar to a cooked cake. In an airtight container or well wrapped in the fridge, this cake will keep for up to 5 days. Perfect with a cup of tea.

SERVES 6–8

Preparation time 20 minutes + standing time

140 g (5 oz/1 cup) walnut pieces
750 g (1 lb 10 oz) carrots, peeled and roughly chopped
125 g (4½ oz/1¼ cups) almond meal (see Note)
245 g (8¾ oz/1½ cups) fresh pitted dates
¼ teaspoon ground nutmeg
2 teaspoons ground cinnamon
1 teaspoon ground ginger
90 g (3¼ oz/1 cup) desiccated coconut
4 tablespoons sultanas
1 quantity Labne (page 27)
2 tablespoons maple syrup

Chop the walnuts for **3 sec/speed 4**. Remove and set aside.

Grate the carrot for **20 sec/speed 8**. Transfer to a clean tea towel and squeeze out as much excess liquid as possible. (Save the juice for drinking later!)

Blend the almond meal, dates, spices and a pinch of sea salt for **10 sec/speed 4** until the mixture sticks together. Add the carrot, coconut, sultanas and most of the walnuts. Mix for **1 min/speed 2**.

Double line a 15 cm (6 in) springform cake tin with plastic wrap. Firmly press the mixture into the tin, ensuring there are no air pockets. Chill in the fridge for at least 1 hour.

Combine the labne and maple syrup in a bowl to make a frosting. Remove the cake from the tin, then spread over the frosting. Scatter over the remaining walnuts to serve.

MAKE AHEAD: FRIDGE
GLUTEN-FREE | VEGETARIAN

NOTE

One of the great joys of being a thermo owner is having the ability to mill your own flours and meals. Make your own almond meal by milling the same weight in blanched almonds for **15 sec/ speed 10***. It's simple and more nutritious.*

NUTTERTELLA MOUSSE

CHOCOLATE TRUFFLES

This vegan mousse tastes even better than the unhealthier original, which is laden with cream and eggs. I like to serve these in little glass jars, but you can easily serve it from one large container, if you prefer. This keeps in the fridge for up to 5 days.

SERVES 4

Preparation time 5 minutes + standing time

1 quantity Nuttertella (page 21)
140 ml (4¾ fl oz) coconut cream
½ ripe avocado, stone removed, peeled
1 tablespoon raw cacao powder, plus extra to serve
coconut flakes (optional), to serve

Blend all of the ingredients for **20 sec/ speed 8**.

Divide the mixture evenly between four small serving glasses or jars.

Place in the fridge to set for at least 6 hours, or preferably overnight.

Serve with coconut flakes, if using, and some cacao powder sprinkled on top.

MAKE AHEAD: FRIDGE

DAIRY-FREE | GLUTEN-FREE | PALEO | VEGAN | VEGETARIAN | LOW-CARB

These soft and absolutely delicious little balls of goodness require very little effort. Coconut oil melts at 24°C (75°F), so depending on the weather, you may need to refrigerate the mixture for about 30 minutes before rolling into balls. Pop them straight back in to chill once they've been rolled. If the coconut oil separates from the mixture, just work it in with your hands as you roll. Store these in an airtight container in the fridge for up 2 weeks.

MAKES 22

Preparation time 25 minutes + standing time

1 quantity Nuttertella (page 21)
2 tablespoons raw cacao powder
3 tablespoons coconut oil
35 g (1¼ oz/½ cup) unsweetened shredded coconut

Blend the nuttertella, 1 tablespoon of the cacao powder and coconut oil for **10 sec/speed 4**.

Roll the mixture into 2.5 cm (1 in) balls, then place in the fridge for 30 minutes, or until firm.

Chop the shredded coconut in the clean mixer bowl for **2 min/120°C/speed 2**. Add the remaining cacao powder and blend for **10 sec/ speed 5**. Transfer this mixture to a shallow dish or bowl.

Roll the truffles in the coconut mixture to coat, pressing it into the surface. Refrigerate.

MAKE AHEAD: FRIDGE

DAIRY-FREE | GLUTEN-FREE | VEGAN | VEGETARIAN

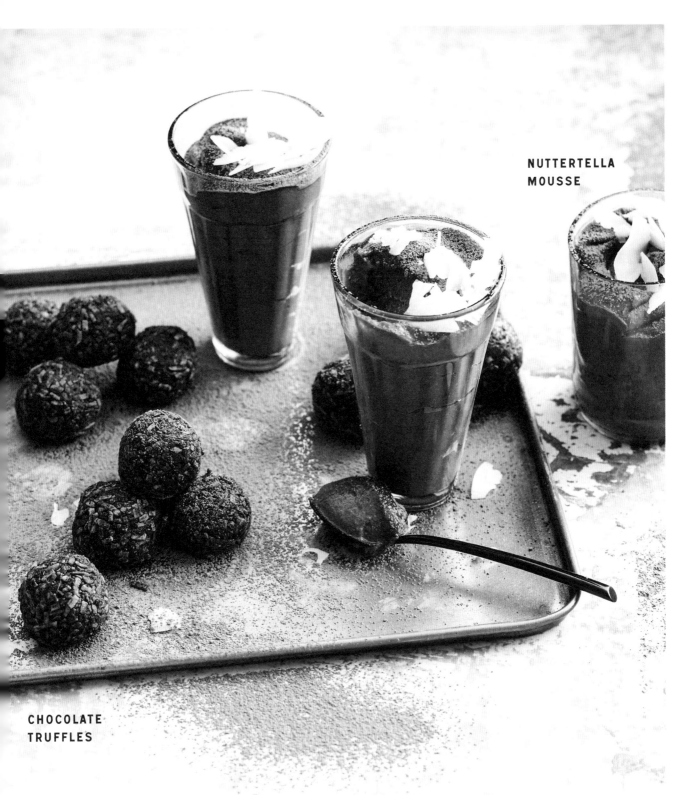

NUTTERTELLA
MOUSSE

CHOCOLATE
TRUFFLES

FIGGY BROWN RICE PUDDING AND MAPLE MACADAMIA CRUNCH

I like to use macadamia milk for this recipe because macadamias have a higher fat content, making the milk extra creamy. You could also use coconut or soy milk, if you didn't want to use nut milk. Quinoa can also be swapped for the brown rice, just follow the soaking instructions on page 97. I always make a triple batch of the maple macadamia crunch because it's such an easy way to add a crunchy topping to desserts (or porridge, if your morning needs a little lift!).

SERVES 4

Preparation time 5 minutes
Cooking time 30 minutes

Maple macadamia crunch
4 tablespoons macadamias, roughly chopped
3 tablespoons maple syrup

Brown rice pudding
8 dried figs, halved, plus extra to serve
1 litre (35 fl oz/4 cups) macadamia milk or other nut milk (page 43)
220 g (7¾ oz/1 cup) brown rice
1 vanilla bean, split and seeds scraped (optional)
3 tablespoons black chia seeds (optional)

Cook the macadamias, maple syrup and a pinch of sea salt for **5 min/120°C/reverse stir/speed 2**. Transfer to a bowl and set aside. Don't wash the bowl.

Chop the figs for **10 sec/speed 4**. Scrape down the side of the bowl. Add the milk and rice, and the vanilla and chia seeds, if using. Cook for **25 min/90°C/reverse stir/speed 2**, or until the rice is tender.

Serve the rice pudding immediately with the maple macadamia crunch and a few dried figs on top.

DAIRY-FREE | GLUTEN-FREE | VEGAN | VEGETARIAN

PISTACHIO AND CARDAMOM KULFI

Cashews, almonds, macadamias, or even a combination of nuts can also be used in this recipe. But I prefer using pistachios for a more traditional flavour, and also because I just love them! When making the nut milk for this recipe, follow the recipe on page 43, but blend the nuts with 750 ml (26 fl oz/3 cups) of water rather than a litre.

MAKES APPROXIMATELY 1 LITRE (35 FL OZ/4 CUPS)

Preparation time 5 minutes + standing time
Cooking time 25 minutes

750 ml (26 fl oz/3 cups) pistachio milk (see recipe introduction),
    reserving pistachio meal
400 ml (14 fl oz) tin coconut cream
175 g (6 oz/½ cup) raw honey
2 teaspoons ground cardamom
2 teaspoons gluten-free cornflour (cornstarch)
crushed pistachios, to serve (optional)

Add all of the ingredients to the mixer bowl including the pistachio meal and blend for **10 sec/speed 4**.

Attach the simmering basket, instead of the measuring cup, to the mixer bowl lid. Cook for **25 min/90°C/speed 3**.

Pour the mixture into popsicle moulds or a 1 litre (35 fl oz/4 cup) container. Place in the freezer for at least 4 hours, or until firm.

Let the kulfi stand for 10–15 minutes to soften slightly before serving.

Serve with crushed pistachios.

See photograph on page 186.

MAKE AHEAD: FREEZE
DAIRY-FREE | GLUTEN-FREE | VEGETARIAN

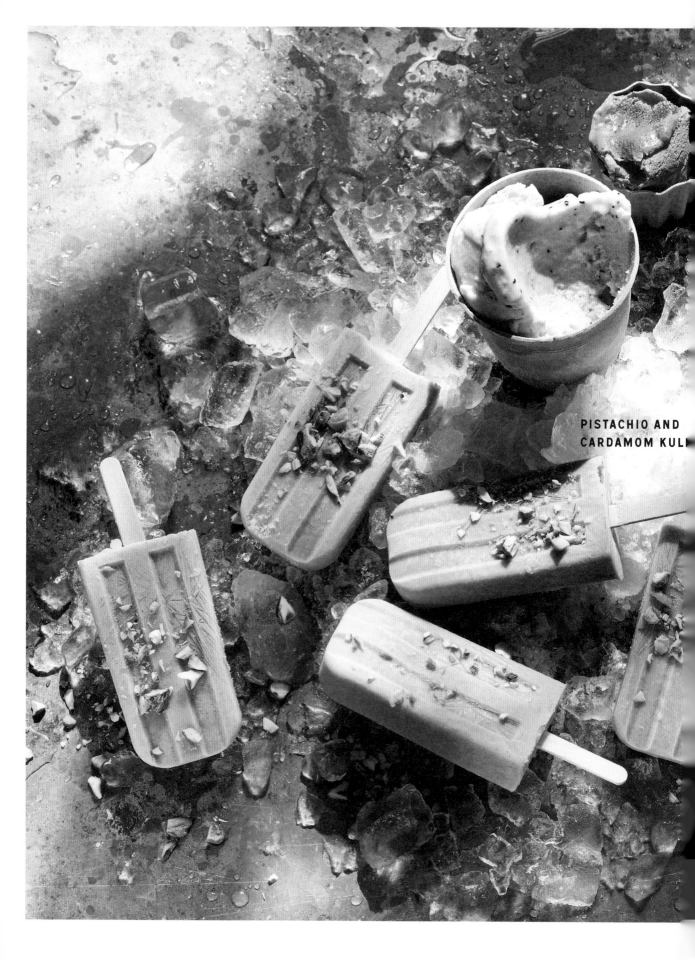

PISTACHIO AND
CARDAMOM KUL

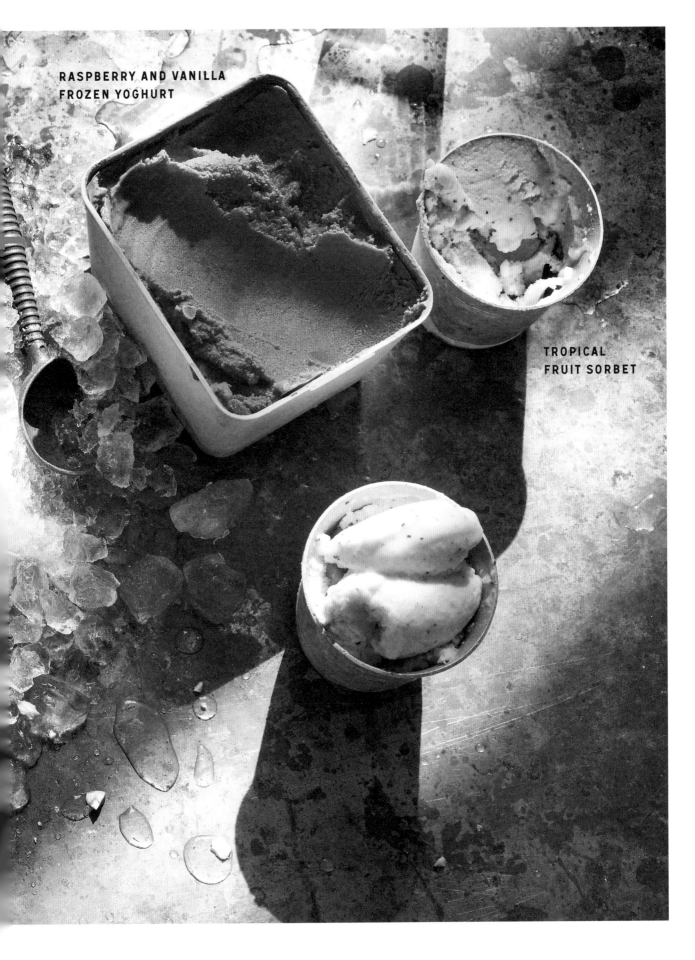

RASPBERRY AND VANILLA
FROZEN YOGHURT

TROPICAL
FRUIT SORBET

TROPICAL FRUIT SORBET

This is a back-to-front sorbet: instead of churning and waiting for it to freeze, you freeze first then blend and devour. You can easily change it up with other tropical fruits like mango, papaya, stone fruits or banana if you want to make a few different versions during the warmer months. Be sure to taste how sweet your mixture is before you add the syrup. Your fruit may have enough sweetness. You can also make popsicles with this mixture. If you are not eating it straight away, it will need a little longer than usual to soften before eating.

MAKES APPROXIMATELY 750 ML (26 FL OZ/3 CUPS)
Preparation time 10 minutes + standing time

400 g (14 oz) peeled and cored ripe pineapple, roughly chopped
560 g (1 lb 4 oz) tinned lychees, drained
pulp from 2 passionfruit
1 tablespoon lime juice
1 tablespoon rice syrup or maple syrup (optional)
1 x 270 ml (9½ fl oz) tin coconut cream

Blend all of the ingredients and a pinch of sea salt for **10 sec/speed 6**. Transfer the mixture to a shallow container and place in the freezer for 4 hours, or until firm.

Add the mixture to the mixer bowl, breaking it up into large chunks if possible to help it blend more easily. Turn on the mixer, gradually increasing to **speed 8/1–2 min** until the ice crystals have completely broken down and the mixture is smooth.

Insert the whisk attachment for **20 sec/speed 4**. Serve immediately, or return to the freezer for 1 hour to firm up slightly.

See photograph on page 187.

MAKE AHEAD: FREEZE
DAIRY-FREE | GLUTEN-FREE | NUT-FREE | VEGAN | VEGETARIAN

RASPBERRY AND VANILLA FROZEN YOGHURT

Frozen yoghurt has had a place in my heart from a young age. Back in my school days, you could buy processed yoghurt in tubs – those had a whole lot of sugar and not much yoghurt (but I still loved the taste). There is rarely ice cream in the freezer in our house, but this frozen yoghurt always makes the cut. I love the tartness of the raspberries and yoghurt with the sweetness of the vanilla and maple syrup, but feel free to change the fruit. Mango or peach frozen yoghurt are also delicious.

MAKES APPROXIMATELY 750 G (1 LB 10 OZ)

Preparation time 10 minutes + standing time

500 g (1 lb 2 oz) Homemade goat's yoghurt (page 26), or cow's yoghurt
2 teaspoons vanilla bean paste or natural vanilla extract
3 tablespoons maple syrup
250 g (9 oz) frozen raspberries

Combine the yoghurt, vanilla, maple syrup and a pinch of sea salt in a shallow container and place in the freezer for 4 hours, or until firm.

Add the frozen yoghurt and the frozen raspberries to the mixer bowl, breaking things up into chunks, if possible, to help it blend more easily. Turn on the mixer, gradually increasing to **speed 8/1–2 min** until the ice crystals have completely broken down and the mixture is smooth.

Insert the whisk attachment for **20 sec/speed 4**. Serve immediately, or return to the freezer for 1 hour to firm up slightly.

See photograph on page 187.

MAKE AHEAD: FREEZE
GLUTEN-FREE | NUT-FREE | VEGETARIAN

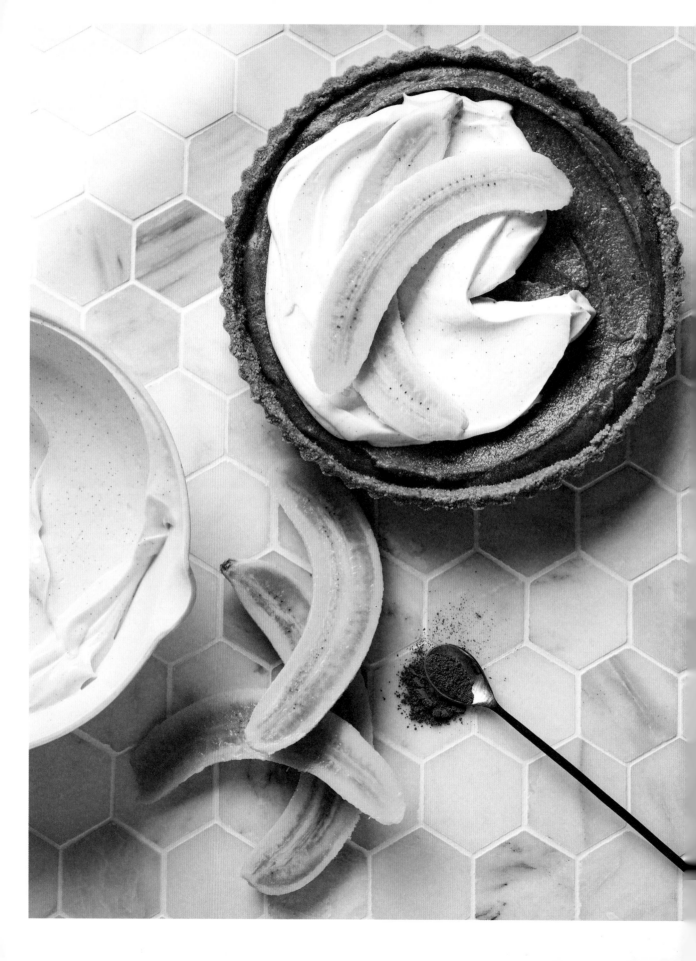

BANOFFEE CHEESECAKE (AKA 'THE SILENCER')

I call this 'cheesecake' The Silencer because whenever I serve it, there is total silence around the table as every last crumb is scoffed down. It is so easy to throw together, and you can use any old pie tin – it doesn't have to be fluted.

SERVES 6

Preparation time 20 minutes + standing time
Cooking time 1 minute

200 g (7 oz) plain, crumbly sweet biscuits, such as digestives
100 g (3½ oz) coconut oil
1 quantity Vegan salted caramel sauce (page 51)
5 bananas, halved lengthways
1 quantity Labne (page 27)
1 teaspoon vanilla bean paste or natural vanilla extract
2 tablespoons maple syrup
ground cinnamon, to serve

Chop the biscuits for **5 sec/speed 6**. Add the coconut oil and cook for **1 min/60°C/speed 2**.

Transfer the mixture to a 22 cm (8½ in) fluted loose-based tart (flan) tin. Evenly and firmly press the mixture into the tin, then refrigerate until needed.

Blend the caramel sauce and 2 of the bananas for **30 sec/speed 6** until well combined. Spoon all of the mixture into the cake base, spread around evenly and return to the fridge to firm up for about 4 hours, or overnight.

Blend the labne, vanilla and maple syrup for **15 sec/speed 5**. Spread the cheese mixture over the caramel filling. Top with the remaining banana halves and sprinkle with cinnamon before serving.

NUT-FREE | VEGETARIAN

MANGO AND COCONUT STICKY RICE

I've visited Thailand many times, and when there I make it my mission to grab a little bowl of mango sticky rice from a street stall. Before my thermo-loving days, I found this dessert too much of a hassle to prepare at home. Now I can recreate it whenever I like, and I still can't believe it's this simple.

SERVES 4

Preparation time 10 minutes + standing time
Cooking time 35 minutes

300 g (10½ oz/1½ cups) white glutinous rice, plus 1 teaspoon extra
270 ml (9½ fl oz) tin coconut cream
125 ml (4 fl oz/½ cup) rice syrup or raw sugar
½ teaspoon fine sea salt
2 mangoes, cheeks removed, thinly sliced
Black Gomasio (page 39) or sesame seeds, to serve (optional)

Soak the 300 g of rice in cold water for at least 4 hours, but preferably overnight. Drain the rice well in the simmering basket then rinse it under running water until the water coming out of the basket is running clear.

Add 500 g (1 lb 2 oz) of water to the mixer bowl. Insert the simmering basket into the mixer bowl. Shape the rice into a mound. Cook for **25–30 min/steam mode/speed 2** until the rice is tender. Remove the simmering basket and cover with a tea towel to keep the rice warm. Drain the water from the mixer bowl, then dry it completely.

Mill the extra teaspoon of rice for **40 sec/speed 10**. Add the coconut cream, rice syrup and salt to the milled rice. Cook for **5 min/100°C/speed 1**, or until the mixture is nice and thick.

Spoon 4 tablespoons of this coconut cream mixture into a bowl and set aside. Insert the whisk attachment, then add the warm rice to the rest of the coconut cream. Mix for **1 min/speed 1** until very well combined. Set aside in the mixer bowl for 10 minutes to allow the rice to absorb the coconut cream mixture.

Serve the sticky rice topped with the sliced mango, a generous drizzle of the reserved coconut cream and a sprinkle of gomasio.

DAIRY-FREE | GLUTEN-FREE | VEGAN | VEGETARIAN

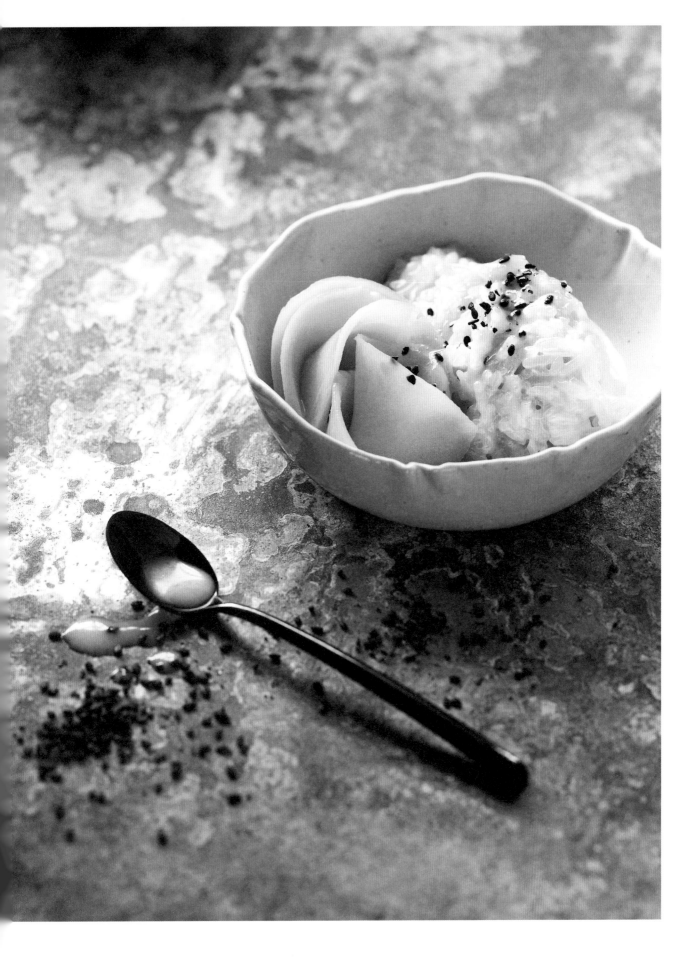

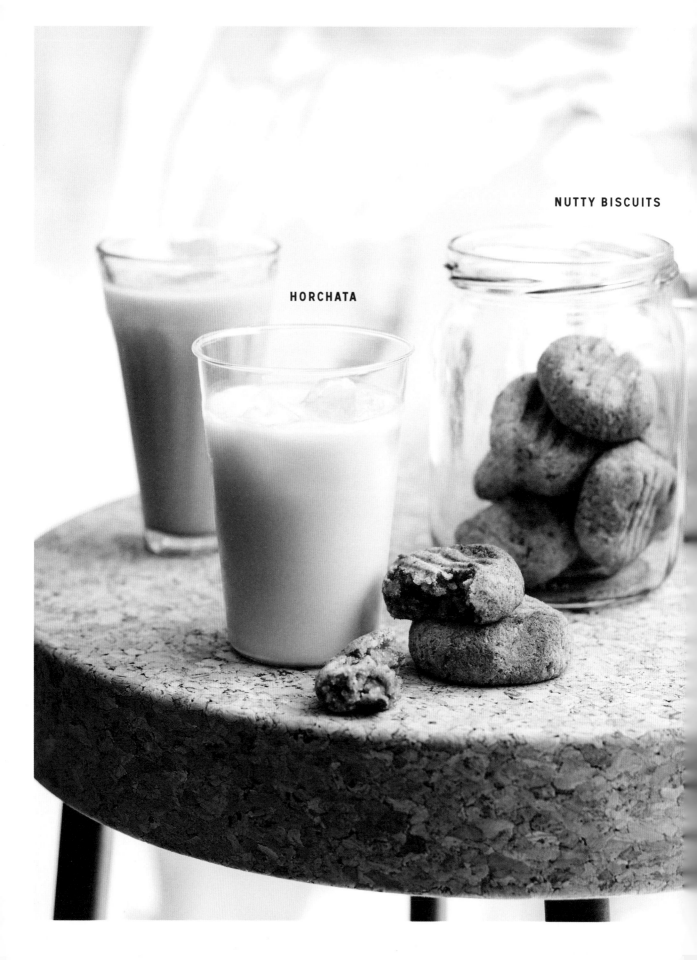

HORCHATA

NUTTY BISCUITS

HORCHATA

Horchata is a spiced milky drink found across Latin American countries. It makes a great alternative to those terrible milkshakes made with syrups and who knows what else! Horchata keeps in the fridge for up to 2 days. As it's a natural product, it will separate, but a good stir before serving fixes that.

MAKES APPROXIMATELY 1.5 LITRES (52 FL OZ/6 CUPS)
Preparation time 10 minutes + standing time

80 g (2¾ oz/½ cup) natural almonds
140 g (5 oz/¾ cup) long grain rice
1 cinnamon stick
2 teaspoons sesame seeds
1 vanilla bean, split and seeds scraped or
   1 teaspoon natural vanilla extract
3 tablespoons maple syrup

Place the almonds in a bowl. Cover completely with lukewarm water and add a good pinch of salt. Cover with a tea towel and set aside to soak for 8 hours.

Drain the almonds in a sieve and rinse well under plenty of running water. Blend the rice and cinnamon for **1 min/speed 10**. Add the almonds, vanilla, maple syrup and 1.5 litres (52 fl oz/6 cups) of water and blend for **2 min/speed 9**.

Refrigerate for 4 hours, or overnight. Strain the horchata through a sieve lined with muslin (cheesecloth), or a nut-milk bag, discarding any solids. Keep in the fridge and when ready to serve, stir gently then pour over ice.

MAKE AHEAD: FRIDGE
GLUTEN-FREE | DAIRY-FREE | VEGAN | VEGETARIAN

NUTTY BISCUITS

If you make your own nut milks, all the perfectly good leftover nut meal can be used in these soft and chewy biscuits. Less waste is always good! Harder nuts yield more leftover meal than softer ones. Freeze until you have enough to make these – any combination of nut meals will be delicious.

MAKES 12
Preparation time 10 minutes
Cooking time 15 minutes

1 tablespoon chia seeds
2 tablespoons shredded coconut
120 g (4¼ oz/⅔ cup) fresh dates, pitted
100 g (3½ oz) nut meal (see Tip on
   page 43)
2 tablespoons plain (all-purpose) flour
60 g (2¼ oz) Butter (page 22), melted

Preheat the oven to 180°C (350°F). Line a baking tray with baking paper.

Place the chia seeds in a bowl with 1 tablespoon of water. Soak for 10 minutes.

Meanwhile, chop the coconut and dates for **10 sec/speed 4**. Add the soaked chia seeds, nut meal, flour, melted butter and a pinch of salt. Mix for **1 min/dough mode**.

Roll the mixture into 3 cm (1¼ in) balls and place these 5 cm (2 in) apart on the lined tray. Use a fork to press down and flatten them slightly to about 2 cm (¾ in) thick. Bake for 15 minutes, or until golden.

Set aside to cool completely. Store in an airtight container in the fridge for up to 5 days.

MAKE AHEAD: FRIDGE
VEGETARIAN

THAI COCONUT SHAKE

I can't get enough of icy-cold coconut shakes, in any form.
Although these coconut shakes are great with a good squeeze
of lime juice, it's often the simplest of things that taste the
best. That's why this recipe is all about the coconut. These are
the best thirst quenchers for your family in the summer
months. If you're not confident opening up young coconuts,
use 700 ml (24 fl oz) coconut water (there's about 350 ml/
12 fl oz in a young coconut) and then triple the shredded
coconut. When it comes to sweetness, how much maple syrup
you'll need will depend on your taste, and on how sweet the
coconut water is. Anything thicker than maple syrup doesn't
blend very well.

SERVES 4

Preparation time 10 minutes

2 young coconuts, chilled
405 g (14¼ oz/3 cups) ice cubes
1–2 tablespoons maple syrup (optional)
2 tablespoons shredded coconut (optional)

Carefully crack open the coconuts with a large heavy knife or a cleaver.
Strain the coconut juice through a fine-mesh sieve into the mixer bowl.
Using a spoon, scoop all of the flesh in to the mixer bowl.

Add the remaining ingredients, if using, and blend for **20 sec/speed 10**.

Serve right away.

**DAIRY-FREE | GLUTEN-FREE | NUT-FREE | PALEO | VEGAN |
VEGETARIAN | LOW-CARB**

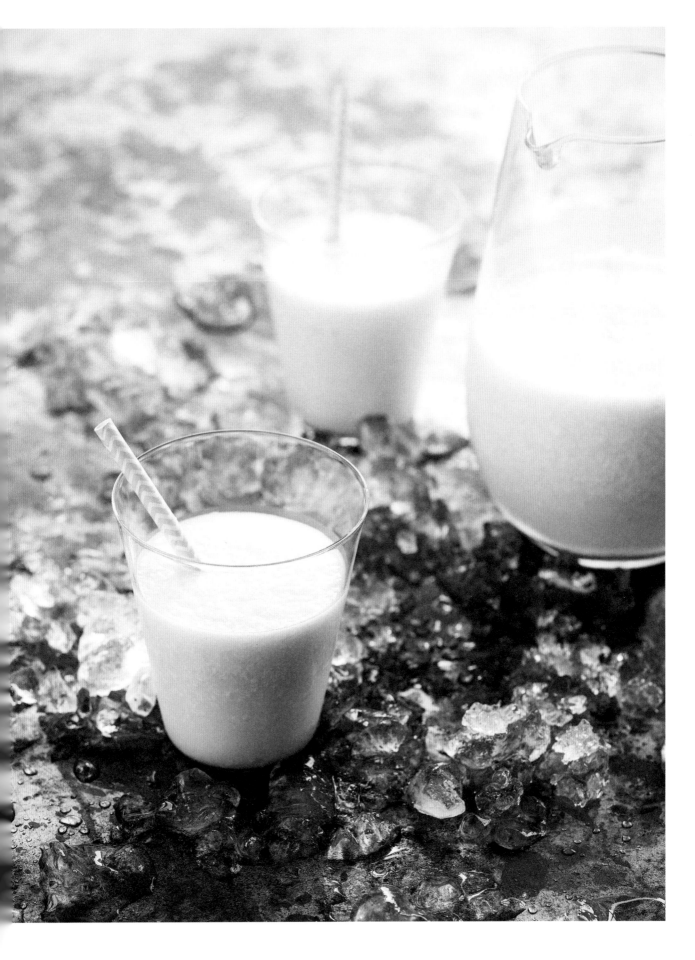

HONEY CINNAMON SCROLLS WITH CREAM CHEESE GLAZE

Let's call this saving the best till last! While the making of these scrolls is definitely a little more involved than the other desserts in this chapter, every bite is worth every minute of effort. And the more you make them, the easier and more enjoyable it gets.

Traditionally, the dough is slathered in cinnamon butter before baking, but using nutter butter is definitely a substitute worth trying. You can't argue with it in terms of benefits and flavour. Who says a healthier version can't beat the original?

MAKES 12

Preparation time 30 minutes + standing time
Cooking time 40 minutes

200 ml (7 fl oz) milk
150 g (5½ oz) Butter (page 22)
1 vanilla bean, split and seeds scraped or 2 teaspoons natural vanilla extract
7 g (⅙ oz/2 teaspoons) dried active yeast
485 g (1 lb 1 oz/3¼ cups) plain (all-purpose) flour, plus extra for dusting
1 egg, plus 1 egg yolk for brushing
175 g (6 oz/½ cup) raw honey
1½ tablespoons ground cinnamon
150 g (5½ oz) Nutter butter (page 21)

Cream cheese glaze
125 ml (4 fl oz/½ cup) maple syrup
¼ teaspoon fine sea salt
3 tablespoons Labne (page 27)

Add the milk, 125 g (4½ oz) of the butter and vanilla to the mixer bowl. Cook for **3–4 min/50°C/speed**, or until the butter melts. Allow the mixture to cool to 37°C (99°F).

Sprinkle the yeast into the milk mixture in the mixer bowl. Mix for **30 sec/soft stir**. Add the flour, egg and 1 tablespoon of the honey. Mix for **8 sec/speed 3**. Scrape down the side of the bowl. Knead for **5 min/dough mode**.

Transfer the dough to a large bowl and cover with a tea towel or plastic wrap. Set aside in a warm, draught-free place for 1 hour, or until the dough has doubled in size.

Meanwhile, put the cinnamon, nutter butter and remaining honey in the mixer bowl and mix for **20 sec/speed 3**. Transfer to a bowl and set aside at room temperature. Wash and dry the mixer bowl.

Punch the dough to knock the air out of it, then transfer to the mixer bowl and knead for **5 min/dough mode**.

Meanwhile, line a large baking tray with baking paper.

Transfer the dough to a lightly floured surface and shape it into a rectangular shape. Use a rolling pin to roll it out to a 1 cm (½ in) thick rectangle, about 40 x 30 cm (16 x 12 in). Spread the cinnamon nutter butter evenly over the top. Carefully and tightly, roll the dough up at the longest edge to make a log shape. Using a sharp knife, cut 12 even-sized pieces. Place the scrolls, cut side up, onto the lined baking tray about 2 cm (¾ in) apart. Cover with a tea towel and set aside in a warm place for a further 30 minutes, or until the scrolls have almost doubled in size.

Preheat the oven to 180°C (350°F). Lightly beat the reserved egg yolk and brush this over the scrolls. Bake in the oven for 20–30 minutes, until golden and cooked. Remove and set aside for 5 minutes while you make the glaze.

Add the maple syrup and salt to the mixer bowl. Cook for **2 min/50°C/ speed 1**. Add the labne and mix for **30 sec/speed 4**.

Drizzle half of the glaze all over the scrolls then set them aside for 5 minutes. Drizzle over the remaining glaze then allow to sit for a few minutes before serving. Keep in an airtight container for 2–3 days.

See photograph on pages 200–1.

TIP

You may need to heat your cinnamon butter very gently to make it spreadable.

VEGETARIAN

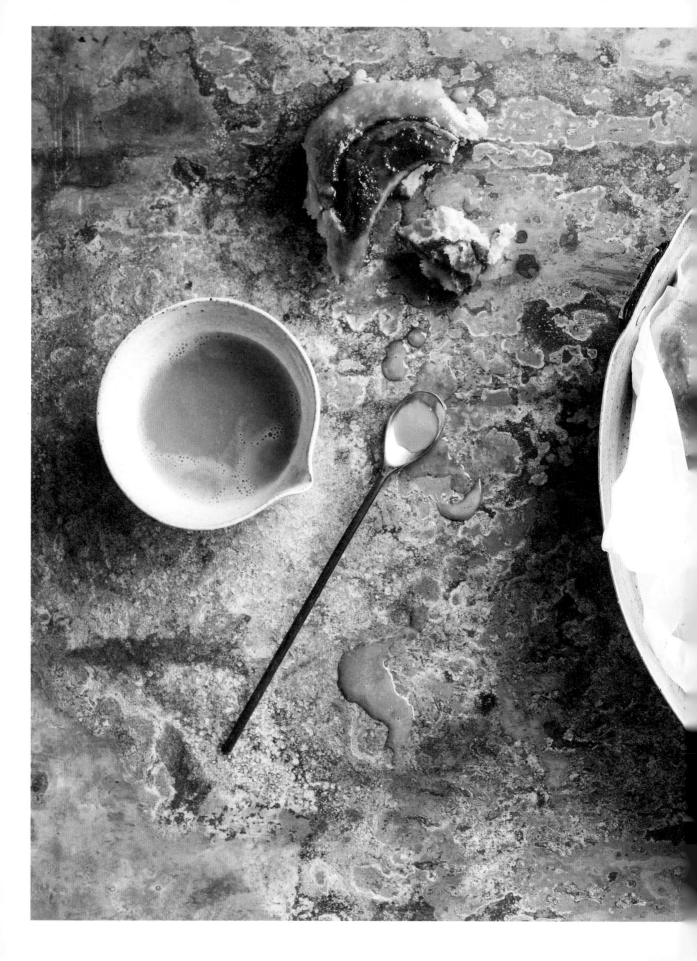

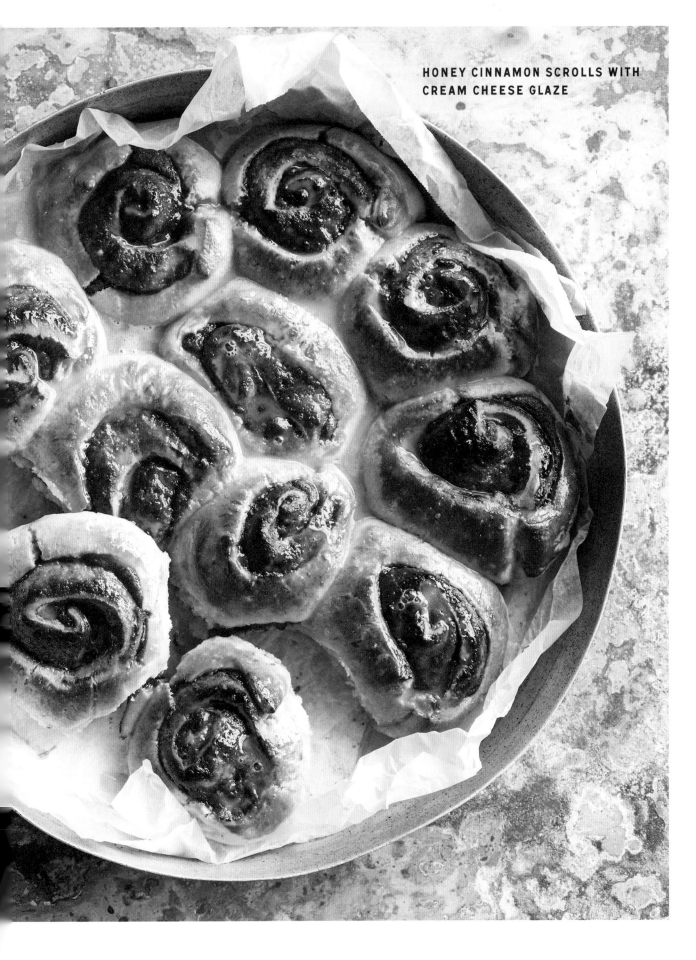

HONEY CINNAMON SCROLLS WITH
CREAM CHEESE GLAZE

INDEX

ABOUT THE AUTHOR

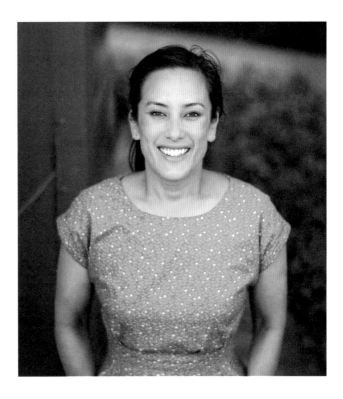

Over the last 12 years, Olivia Andrews has worked as a recipe developer, food writer and stylist for some of Australia's most prestigious food magazines and TV shows, including *delicious, SBS Feast, MasterChef, Destination Flavour* and *The Biggest Loser*. Most recently, she co-founded the hugely popular recipe kit delivery service Marley Spoon, where she continues to inspire families with her easy, flavour-packed approach to weeknight meals. *Healthy Thermo Cooking For Busy Families* is Olivia's second cookbook, following her first health-food title, *Whole Food Slow Cooked*.

PUBLISHED IN 2018 BY MURDOCH BOOKS,
AN IMPRINT OF ALLEN & UNWIN

Murdoch Books Australia
83 Alexander Street
Crows Nest NSW 2065
Phone: +61 (0) 2 8425 0100
Fax: +61 (0) 2 9906 2218
murdochbooks.com.au
info@murdochbooks.com.au

Murdoch Books UK
Ormond House
26–27 Boswell Street
London WC1N 3JZ
Phone: +44 (0) 20 8785 5995
murdochbooks.co.uk
info@murdochbooks.co.uk

For Corporate Orders & Custom Publishing,
contact our Business Development Team at
salesenquiries@murdochbooks.com.au.

Publisher: Jane Morrow
Editorial Manager: Katie Bosher
Design Manager: Vivien Valk
Illustrator: Alissa Dinallo
Photographer: Jeremy Simons
Stylist: David Morgan
Home Economists: Olivia Andrews, Alistair Clarkson,
    Claire Dickson-Smith and Charlie Duffy
Production Director: Lou Playfair

A cataloguing-in-publication entry is available from
the catalogue of the National Library of Australia
at nla.gov.au.
A catalogue record for this book is available from
the British Library.

ISBN 978 1 76063 191 8 Australia
ISBN 978 1 76063 438 4 UK

Colour reproduction by Splitting Image Colour
Studio Pty Ltd, Clayton, Victoria
Printed by C & C Offset Printing Co. Ltd., China

DISCLAIMER: The purchaser of this book understands that the operating information contained within is not intended to replace the thermo appliance instructions supplied by the manufacturer. The author and publisher claim no responsibility to any person or entity for any liability, loss, damage or injury caused or alleged to be caused directly or indirectly as a result of the use, application or interpretation of the material in this book. It is understood that you will carefully follow the safety instructions supplied by the manufacturer before operating your thermo appliance.

IMPORTANT: Those who might be at risk from the effects of salmonella poisoning (the elderly, pregnant women, young children and those suffering from immune deficiency diseases) should consult their doctor with any concerns about eating raw eggs.

OVEN GUIDE: You may find cooking times vary depending on the oven you are using. For fan-forced ovens, as a general rule, set the oven temperature to 20°C (70°F) lower than indicated in the recipe.

MEASURES GUIDE: We have used 20 ml (4 teaspoon) tablespoon measures. If you are using a 15 ml (3 teaspoon) tablespoon add an extra teaspoon of the ingredient for each tablespoon specified.

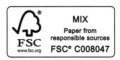

The paper in this book is FSC® certified.
FSC® promotes environmentally responsible,
socially beneficial and economically viable
management of the world's forests.